In Silico Modeling and Simulation for Diabetes Therapy

Authored by

Darshna M. Joshi

Department of Instrumentation and Control Engineering
Government Polytechnic Ahmedabad
Ahmedabad-380015
Gujarat, India

Hardik Bhatt

Department of Pharmaceutical Chemistry
Institute of Pharmacy, Nirma University
Ahmedabad-382481
Gujarat, India

&

Himanshu K. Patel

Department of Electronics and Instrumentation
Institute of Technology, Nirma University
Ahmedabad-382481
Gujarat, India

In Silico Modeling and Simulation for Diabetes Therapy

Authors: Darshna M. Joshi, Hardik Bhatt and Himanshu K. Patel

ISBN (Online): 979-8-89881-363-5

ISBN (Print): 979-8-89881-364-2

ISBN (Paperback): 979-8-89881-365-9

© 2026, Bentham Books imprint.

Published by Bentham Science Publishers Pte. Ltd. Singapore. All Rights Reserved.

First published in 2026.

need for a court order if at any point you breach any terms of this License Agreement. In no event will any delay or failure by Bentham Science Publishers in enforcing your compliance with this License Agreement constitute a waiver of any of its rights.

3. You acknowledge that you have read this License Agreement, and agree to be bound by its terms and conditions. To the extent that any other terms and conditions presented on any website of Bentham Science Publishers conflict with, or are inconsistent with, the terms and conditions set out in this License Agreement, you acknowledge that the terms and conditions set out in this License Agreement shall prevail.

Bentham Science Publishers Pte. Ltd.
No. 9 Raffles Place
Office No. 26-01
Singapore 048619
Singapore
Email: subscriptions@benthamscience.net

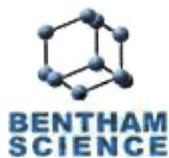

CONTENTS

FOREWORD

"Insulin is not a cure for diabetes; it is a treatment. It enables the diabetic to burn sufficient carbohydrates, so that proteins and fats may be added to the diet in sufficient quantities to provide energy for the economic burdens of life." ~ **Frederick Grant Banting**

Banting, a Canadian pharmacologist, gave the above-mentioned statement back in 1930; however, much has changed over the years. The key to this is "Gene Therapy". This excellent piece of work by Darshna et al. provides a good source of information for readers. Understanding phenotypes and their genetic determinants for diabetes and Metabolic Syndrome (MetS) has been quite challenging. With the advent of systems bioinformatics approaches, there is a need to decipher methods for the identification and evaluation of the functional role of phenotypic traits associated with complex diseases. There are associated phenotypes, such as monogenic syndromes and lipodystrophies, that have been used to understand the molecular pathophysiology of Insulin Resistance (IR) underlying obesity and diabetes mellitus. Consequently, these associated phenotypes have been accompanied by a varied genetic approach, as well as urbanization, globalization, and, of course, changes in food and dietary patterns, in addition to epigenetic spectrums. However, there has been a global shift in dietary patterns, which has driven the upsurge of diet-related non-communicable diseases such as Type 2 Diabetes Mellitus (T2DM) and other diseases such as obesity, Cardiovascular Diseases (CVD), and cancer.

Over the years, researchers have conducted a diverse spectrum of Genome-wide Association Studies (GWAS) associated with T2DM. Several consortia aimed to delineate distinct signals and fine-map the sub-population diversity using multi-ancestry meta-analysis, wherein risk scores are shown to have clinical significance. Intriguingly, Polygenic Risk Scores (PRS) remain key among individuals in correlating disease markers. As an extension to the Genetic Risk Score (GRS), the heritability of mutations serves as a rich resource for gene therapy.

Taken together, there is promise for managing diabetes using *in silico* modeling and simulations. "*In Silico* Modeling and Simulation for Diabetes Therapy" is a resource for scientists, diabetologists, bioinformaticists, genomicists, and, importantly, laymen who need to be educated on data-driven therapy. I congratulate the authors on this wonderful piece.

Long Hail Precision Medicine!

Yours for Science
Prashanth N Suravajhala
Founder, Bioclues.org

PREFACE

The origin of "*In silico* Modeling and Simulation for Diabetes Therapy" stems from a thoughtful commitment to address the challenges and opportunities in diabetes management through *in silico* modeling and computational approaches. This book is designed for a diverse audience, including early-career researchers, trained professionals, and pharmacists who seek to deepen their knowledge of how *in silico* modeling and simulation techniques can boost technological advancements in diabetes. We begin our journey by investigating the fundamentals of how computational tools might help us understand the complexity of diabetes. From there, we look at current technologies and their promising future. In these pages, we highlight not only the technical but also the moral and legal issues that are vital to the proper application of cutting-edge diabetes treatment solutions.

Darshna M. Joshi
Department of Instrumentation and Control Engineering
Government Polytechnic Ahmedabad
Ahmedabad-380015
Gujarat, India

Hardik Bhatt
Department of Pharmaceutical Chemistry
Institute of Pharmacy, Nirma University
Ahmedabad-382481
Gujarat, India

&

Himanshu K. Patel
Department of Electronics and Instrumentation
Institute of Technology, Nirma University
Ahmedabad-382481
Gujarat, India

DEDICATION

This book is dedicated to the persistent pursuit of healing and the hope of a brighter, healthier future. To my parents, whose unwavering love and support have been my guiding light; to my brother, whose encouragement has always been a source of strength; to the Almighty, whose grace has illuminated every step of this journey; and to the readers, whose curiosity and dedication to knowledge fuel progress and inspire change.

ACKNOWLEDGEMENTS

We express our sincere gratitude to the Almighty for granting us the strength, inspiration, and perseverance to bring this work to completion.

Dr. Darshna M. Joshi would like to express her heartfelt gratitude to her parents, Mr. Manojbhai Jayantilal Joshi and Mrs. Bharatiben Manojbhai Joshi, for their unwavering support, encouragement, and blessings throughout her academic journey. Their guidance and belief in the value of education have been a constant source of motivation. She also extends her sincere thanks to her brother, Mr. Parag Manojbhai Joshi, for his encouragement and support.

We gratefully acknowledge the support and academic environment provided by the Directorate of Technical Education, Gujarat, Government Polytechnic Ahmedabad, and Nirma University, which fostered intellectual growth and made it possible to undertake and complete this scholarly work.

We are particularly grateful to Mr. Nikunj Solanki, Photographer at U. N. Mehta Institute of Cardiology & Research Centre, Ahmedabad, for his valuable assistance in editing and formatting the images included in this book. His technical expertise and careful attention to detail significantly enhanced the visual presentation of the material.

We also extend our sincere appreciation to the editorial and production team of Bentham Science Publishers for their guidance, coordination, and support throughout the publication process.

Finally, we thank all individuals who directly or indirectly contributed to the successful completion of this work.

CHAPTER 1

Introduction to *In Silico* Modeling and Simulation

Abstract: Computational advancement is the need of the present century and has played an important role in transforming the medical industry and health research. The application of engineering principles to biology using computational techniques has led to the development of *in silico* modeling and simulation. This chapter discusses the role of computational advancements in medical research and the importance of artificial intelligence and machine learning in modeling and simulation of diseases with personalized healthcare. *In silico* modeling and simulation provide precise predictions about the underlying signaling mechanisms involved in various diseases. This leads to early detection, as well as time-efficient and cost-effective solutions for healthcare practitioners. Computational techniques enhance targeted drug therapy in the pharmaceutical industry, facilitating drug design, development, and testing. Although *in silico* modeling and simulations are trending nowadays, challenges and limitations remain, such as the accuracy of the model, the depth of complex biological models, effective and efficient datasets, the lack of data availability, patient concerns, consent, and finally, the validation of the data as the model persists. Keeping the constraints in mind, the health informatics field has boosted the development and analysis of much more complex models like those related to cancer and diabetes. For advancing the medical industry, the impact of *in silico* models would bring a revolution in patient care. This chapter has attempted to cover everything, from significance to constraints and difficulties in *in silico* modeling.

Keywords: Computational techniques, Disease modeling, Health informatics, *In silico*, Limitations, Medical research, Simulation.

INTRODUCTION

Advancements in computing have been significant over the last 100 years, transforming many industries, including the healthcare system and medical fields. Engineering, biology, and *in silico* methods of modeling and simulation have been developed as a result of the integration of computing tools. It has changed the way diseases are diagnosed, treated, and understood. Health services and physicians are now able to predict medical outcomes, model complex biological systems, and simulate disease processes with the assistance of computation and data tools. This chapter is concerned with the importance of these research tools in medicine and, in particular, how they improve drug development, disease modeling, and personal health management.

Darshna M. Joshi, Hardik Bhatt & Himanshu K. Patel
All rights reserved-© 2026 Bentham Science Publishers

The advancement of computational methods has revolutionized our comprehension of complex biological systems related to various diseases, including cancer, diabetes, and metabolic disorders. Researchers, through *in silico* modeling and simulation, can gain a deep understanding of the molecular signaling pathways of the disease to establish potential biomarkers and therapeutic targets. This significantly increases the chances of disease detection at an early stage, which is important for effective treatment. In addition, these developments provide health professionals with tools that are more efficient in terms of time and cost, allowing them to focus on the quality of care provided to patients.

Detrimental practices have taken over the medical processes of societies, but with the help of technology, there is always a ray of hope. The most critical technologies, AI and ML, have already enabled the innovation of personalized treatments for patients based on their records. There are algorithms designed to scan through various data regions, like clinical records, genetic information, images, and even monitors, allowing for specific treatments to be predicted, alongside making the procedures more accurate. These tools, including AI and ML, have also become essential when it comes to simulating the scope of how a disease is likely to worsen over time and predicting to what extent specific treatments will be helpful. With the advanced healthcare system, patients will now have access to treatments tailored to their specific health conditions and genetic makeup. It is safe to say that AI and ML have truly won the race for personalized healthcare

The way computational modeling has altered the medical sciences field cannot be overstated, especially for the pharmaceutical industry. The processes for discovering new medications have become much faster and cheaper due to the ability to create and trial new drugs using *in silico* models. *In silico* techniques allow the testing of drug efficacy without the need for expensive clinical trials. In addition, these models help develop and refine formulations and dosages to increase the likelihood of success in treating patients. Also, simulating drug action on biological targets provides valuable insights into the modification of existing treatments or the design of new therapeutic agents.

In silico modeling and simulation have their advantages, but there are challenges and limitations that must be addressed. First, it is important to recognize that the accuracy of a particular computational model is dependent on the assumptions made and the underlying data. As previously discussed, biological systems are highly complex, and the assumption that these systems will perform alike, without any discrepancies between predicted and actual results, is overly simplistic. There is a dire lack of data, and the available information is insufficient for the construction of accurate models. There are also ethical dilemmas, such as a patient's right to withhold consent for the use of their health data, as well as the confidentiality of the information, when applying these computational techniques to medical research. Lastly, there are challenges in confirming models against experimental data, as models are sometimes built on assumptions that overly simplify biological complexities.

The barriers are real, but one cannot dismiss the impact of advancements in computation on medical research. The most challenging diseases are modeled and understood with complete ease now. The development of drugs has become considerably faster, and so has the availability of targeted treatment strategies. This chapter discusses these advancements, their impact, and the hurdles to achieving them in the industry.

ROLE OF COMPUTATIONAL ADVANCEMENTS IN MEDICAL RESEARCH

The combination of medicine, engineering, and interdisciplinary fields leads to the advancement of computational biology. It uses computational methods in engineering to represent and analyze complex biological mechanisms. Various diseases are modeled, and predictions about the target therapies needed to solve complex biological phenomena are made using computational advancements [1, 2]. The advancement in computational methods has shown proven improvement in the understanding of biological systems by healthcare researchers and computational scientists. As per the latest trends, advanced computational methods like Artificial Intelligence (AI)-based machine learning have successfully demonstrated the predictions about sensitive targets for drug therapy, as well as early detection of diseases, which can help manage the biological issues worldwide [1 - 7].

Previously, the diagnosis-to-treatment cycle of any disease was a costly and time-consuming affair. Because of the same, mortality rates have always been higher. Today, metabolic disorders like cancer and diabetes are ruling the world and spreading at a higher speed on a large scale. Early prediction and early diagnosis have become the need of the hour for this purpose. As a result, computational advancements are the best options. Medical diagnostic systems based on computational methods can offer cost-effective and speedy solutions, as well as predictions regarding a certain medical condition. We can harness the power of computational tools, data analysis software, and algorithms to revolutionize the medical research field with early detection, targeted therapy, and drug development, thereby advancing patient healthcare [1, 8 - 11].

Biomedical computation has several roles to play, thanks to its ability to handle and analyze vast amounts of sensitive health-related data. Bytes of data are generated daily, which are handled by the medical researchers, and various useful insights are obtained. Biomedical computation offers sophisticated algorithms to process and derive meaningful insights from this data, enabling the identification of genetic markers, disease pathways, and potential drug targets.

Apart from the data regarding drug therapies and disease predictions, a very important role that computational advancements play is the design and development of medical devices. Medical sensors, 3D tissue, and organ structures have become possible due to the advancement of computational technologies. Digital models of the heart and various other organs have revolutionized the field of medicine. Even surgeries can be planned based on the data received from the medical history of patients [2, 7, 12 - 16].

Despite the limitless role of computational advancements, the challenges faced throughout the process cannot be ignored. Overall, computational methods can be used to provide health-related information to clinicians, researchers, and pharmacists for the advancement of technologies in the medical field. This chapter discusses the importance, limitations, and uncertainties of *in silico* modeling and simulation. *In silico* modeling refers to the use of computer-based models and simulations for the analysis of complex biological processes. This was previously carried out using *in vivo* and *in vitro* approaches.

In silico and computational modeling are closely related and hence used interchangeably. Below is the list of roles of computational modeling in medical research.

1. Disease modeling and simulations [1].
2. Big data analysis from various health records, as well as real-time data [2].
3. Integration of large amounts of data sets [5].
4. Analysis of genetic-based data for best disease identification and prediction [2].
5. Identification of drug targets [5].
6. Drug design [6] [7].
7. Providing personalized healthcare [9].
8. Assisting disease diagnosis and treatment [9].
9. Analysing biological networks [10].
10. Health informatics [17].
11. Ensuring the safety and security of health data [18].

The above roles are being played by computational advancements in medical research these days, which have provided cost and time-effective solutions for the healthcare industry.

IMPORTANCE OF *IN SILICO* MODELING

An area of biology that focuses on computer-based simulation is *in silico*. It provides very precise predictions regarding the behavior of biological systems, which can later be verified in *in vivo* and *in vitro* analysis carried out in laboratory clinical trials [19]. *In silico* modeling and simulation have gained much attention in the healthcare industry, leading to the optimization of costs and a reduction in animal sacrifices on a larger scale. *In silico* methods are useful at any level, from genetic to detailed, based on data availability. The structure of various molecules can be studied, and modifications can be planned to use various machine learning algorithms and other advancements [20 - 27].

If detailed mechanisms regarding the signaling pathways need to be analyzed, *in silico* modeling would provide a revolutionary platform. For various diseases in the world, *in silico* modeling can be carried out, and the effects of drugs and alternative therapies can be tested. The results will help us find the optimized drug dosage as well as drug targets. It will even boost drug design and drug discovery [28 - 30]. Fig. (**1**) shows the importance of *in silico* modeling in biological research, which includes cost-effectiveness, predictability, drug discovery, time efficiency, and reduction in clinical trials.

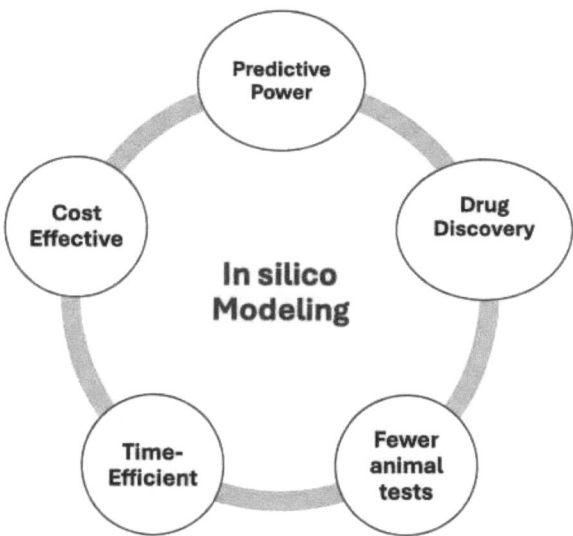

Fig. (1). Importance of *in silico* modeling.

Moreover, *in silico* methods play an important role in modeling various molecular structures, along with their interactions with different receptors. The potential binding between ligands and receptor complexes can provide useful information to identify drug targets. Various simulators have been developed that can model the behavior of diseases like cancer and diabetes, providing outcomes that can be used in animal trials. One such model is presented by Darshna *et al.* [28, 29], where type 2 diabetes is modeled and the effect of alternative therapies like exercise and oleuropein is analyzed. In further chapters, we will focus specifically on the *in silico* modeling and simulation methods for diabetes therapies.

Studies obtained from *in silico* modeling can enhance the understanding of mechanisms that have been unravelled so far. The importance of *in silico* modeling is manifold for the scientific community and medical practitioners. The number of reviews using *in silico* modeling has increased, as this addresses the ethical concerns, carries out critical evaluation, and provides evidence-based outcomes. The only concern is the availability of the dataset. The collection and management of large datasets is a significant concern that needs to be taken care of while dealing with *in silico* studies. The identification of new targets will be utilized by the pharmaceutical industry for the development of drugs, and health researchers can use it to test the effects of alternative therapies on various diseases [31 - 36]. This book aims to conceptualize the importance of *in silico* modeling and simulation, specifically for diabetes. A simple workflow for the development of an *in silico* model is shown in Table **1** [37].

Table 1. Workflow of *in silico* model development [37].

Step	Purpose	Example in Diabetes Research
Define Objectives	Identify the biological process or drug target to study.	Model insulin signaling pathway to understand glucose uptake in T2DM.
Collect Data	Gather biological, genetic, or pharmacological data.	Use insulin receptor binding data or glucose metabolism profiles.
Select Computational Tools	Choose software for modeling and analysis.	Employ MATLAB, COPASI, or Cell Designer for simulations.
Build Model	Create a computational model of the biological system.	Develop a pharmacophore model for receptor agonists.
Simulate and Analyze	Run simulations to test hypotheses or predict outcomes.	Perform molecular docking to study insulin-receptor interactions.
Validate Results	Compare model outputs with experimental data.	Validate glucose uptake predictions with clinical trial results.
Refine and Apply	Adjust the model based on findings and apply it to drug design or therapy.	Optimize inhibitors for better glucose excretion.

LIMITATIONS AND UNCERTAINTIES OF *IN SILICO* TECHNIQUES

Despite the advancements of powerful *in silico* techniques, limitations exist. *In silico* models are often simplified, thereby ignoring complexities in signaling mechanisms, which affects accuracy. The lack of sufficient datasets results in questionable predictions. Computational power constraints limit model expansion and data accessibility. Validation challenges persist; without experimental validation, discrepancies arise. Overfitting of the model on new datasets generates errors. Integrating *in silico* models with experimental data is challenging, impacting result reliability. Ethical and regulatory concerns also create uncertainties in *in silico* techniques [34, 37 - 39].

CONCLUDING REMARKS

A merger of engineering with biological principles has profoundly transformed the field of healthcare by providing extensive support for disease diagnosis and prediction, as well as drug development. Through advanced computational techniques like machine learning and artificial intelligence, healthcare researchers can provide data for better diagnosis of patients. Using *in silico* modeling, we can now model complex biological signaling mechanisms, disease conditions, and ligand-receptor interactions and hence predict the behavior of the drug to provide personalized healthcare. Through this evolution, time and cost-effective solutions are possible in the healthcare industry, which plays a crucial role in dealing with the rise of diseases like cancer and diabetes. *In silico* modeling has emerged as a valuable tool for testing hypotheses and thus enhancing the understanding of complex biological mechanisms for targeted novel therapies. It is conducted before the costly and time-consuming *in vivo and in vitro* experiments. Although technology has advanced, challenges such as the accuracy of the model, the lack of data availability, the oversimplification of the model, computational power, and validation must be addressed to fully use the potential of computational biology. With evolving fields, a powerful interdisciplinary approach will be key to advancing medical research in the modern medical world, while considering limitations and uncertainties to ensure an effective solution.

CONSENT FOR PUBLICATION

We hereby give consent for publication.

REFERENCES

[1]   Sleeman B, Jones P. Computational and mathematical methods in medicine. Comput Math Methods Med 2006; 7(1): 1-2.
[http://dx.doi.org/10.1080/10273660600818264] [PMID: 21812577]

[2]   Stead WW, Lin HS. *Computational technology for effective health care: Immediate steps and strategic*

directions. 2009.
[http://dx.doi.org/10.17226/12572]

[3]   Qureshi R, Irfan M, Ali H, *et al.* Artificial intelligence and biosensors in healthcare and its clinical relevance: A review. IEEE Access 2023; 11: 61600-20.
[http://dx.doi.org/10.1109/ACCESS.2023.3285596]

[4]   Galizzi JP, Lockhart BP, Bril A. Applying systems biology in drug discovery and development. dmdi 2013; 28(2): 67-78.
[http://dx.doi.org/10.1515/dmdi-2013-0002] [PMID: 23612649]

[5]   Claus BL, Underwood DJ. Discovery informatics: its evolving role in drug discovery. Drug Discov Today 2002; 7(18): 957-66.
[http://dx.doi.org/10.1016/S1359-6446(02)02433-9] [PMID: 12546870]

[6]   Augen J. The evolving role of information technology in the drug discovery process. Drug Discov Today 2002; 7(5): 315-23.
[http://dx.doi.org/10.1016/S1359-6446(02)02173-6] [PMID: 11854055]

[7]   Choudhuri S, Yendluri M, Poddar S, *et al.* Recent advancements in computational drug design algorithms through machine learning and optimization. Kinases and Phosphatases 2023; 1(2): 117-40.
[http://dx.doi.org/10.3390/kinasesphosphatases1020008]

[8]   Bian Q, Cahan P. Computational tools for stem cell biology. Trends Biotechnol 2016; 34(12): 993-1009.
[http://dx.doi.org/10.1016/j.tibtech.2016.05.010] [PMID: 27318512]

[9]   Fong SS. Computational approaches to metabolic engineering utilizing systems biology and synthetic biology. Comput Struct Biotechnol J 2014; 11(18): 28-34.
[http://dx.doi.org/10.1016/j.csbj.2014.08.005] [PMID: 25379141]

[10]   Lubiana T, Lopes R, Medeiros P, *et al.* Ten quick tips for harnessing the power of ChatGPT in computational biology. PLOS Comput Biol 2023; 19(8): e1011319.
[http://dx.doi.org/10.1371/journal.pcbi.1011319] [PMID: 37561669]

[11]   Way GP, Greene CS, Carninci P, *et al.* A field guide to cultivating computational biology. PLoS Biol 2021; 19(10): e3001419.
[http://dx.doi.org/10.1371/journal.pbio.3001419] [PMID: 34618807]

[12]   Korthauer K, Kimes PK, Duvallet C, *et al.* A practical guide to methods controlling false discoveries in computational biology. Genome Biol 2019; 20(1): 118.
[http://dx.doi.org/10.1186/s13059-019-1716-1] [PMID: 31164141]

[13]   Fedorov AK, Gelfand MS. Towards practical applications in quantum computational biology. Nature Computational Science 2021; 1(2): 114-9.
[http://dx.doi.org/10.1038/s43588-021-00024-z] [PMID: 38217223]

[14]   Marshall SF, Burghaus R, Cosson V, *et al.* Good practices in model-informed drug discovery and development: Practice, application, and documentation. CPT Pharmacometrics Syst Pharmacol 2016; 5(3): 93-122.
[http://dx.doi.org/10.1002/psp4.12049] [PMID: 27069774]

[15]   Choudhuri S, Mallik S, Ghosh B, *et al.* A review of computational learning and IoT applications to high-throughput array-based sequencing and medical imaging data in drug discovery and other health care systems. In: Applied Smart Health Care Informatics. 2022.
[http://dx.doi.org/10.1002/9781119743187.ch5]

[16]   Wang K, Ho CC, Zhang C, Wang B. A review on the 3D printing of functional structures for medical phantoms and regenerated tissue and organ applications. Engineering (Beijing) 2017; 3(5): 653-62.
[http://dx.doi.org/10.1016/J.ENG.2017.05.013]

[17]   Searls DB. A new online computational biology curriculum. PLOS Comput Biol 2014; 10(6): e1003662.

[http://dx.doi.org/10.1371/journal.pcbi.1003662] [PMID: 24921255]

[18]   Patterson EA, Whelan MP. A framework to establish credibility of computational models in biology. Prog Biophys Mol Biol 2017; 129: 13-9.
[http://dx.doi.org/10.1016/j.pbiomolbio.2016.08.007] [PMID: 27702656]

[19]   Aamer Mehmood M. Use of bioinformatics tools in different spheres of life sciences. J Data Mining Genomics Proteomics 2014; 5(2)
[http://dx.doi.org/10.4172/2153-0602.1000158]

[20]   Behbahani M, Nosrati M, Moradi M, Mohabatkar H. Using Chou's general pseudo amino acid composition to classify laccases from bacterial and fungal sources *via* Chou's five-step rule. Appl Biochem Biotechnol 2020; 190(3): 1035-48.
[http://dx.doi.org/10.1007/s12010-019-03141-8] [PMID: 31659712]

[21]   Mohabatkar H, Ebrahimi S, Moradi M. Using Chou's five-steps rule to classify and predict glutathione s-transferases with different machine learning algorithms and pseudo amino acid composition. Int J Pept Res Ther 2021; 27(1): 309-16.
[http://dx.doi.org/10.1007/s10989-020-10087-7]

[22]   Vellido A. The importance of interpretability and visualization in machine learning for applications in medicine and health care. Neural Comput Appl 2020; 32(24): 18069-83.
[http://dx.doi.org/10.1007/s00521-019-04051-w]

[23]   Nabati F, Moradi M, Mohabatkar H. *In silico* analyzing the molecular interactions of plant-derived inhibitors against E6AP, p53, and c-Myc binding sites of HPV type 16 E6 oncoprotein. Mol Biol Res Commun 2020; 9(2): 71-82.
[http://dx.doi.org/10.22099/mbrc.2020.36522.1483] [PMID: 32802901]

[24]   Sadeghi M, Moradi M, Madanchi H, Johari B. *In silico* study of garlic (*Allium sativum* L.)-derived compounds molecular interactions with α-glucosidase. *In Silico* Pharmacol 2021; 9(1): 11.
[http://dx.doi.org/10.1007/s40203-020-00072-9] [PMID: 33457179]

[25]   Haghighi O, Moradi M. *In Silico* study of the structure and ligand interactions of alcohol dehydrogenase from *Cyanobacterium synechocystis* Sp. PCC 6803 as a Key Enzyme for Biofuel Production. Appl Biochem Biotechnol 2020; 192(4): 1346-67.
[http://dx.doi.org/10.1007/s12010-020-03400-z] [PMID: 32767175]

[26]   Haghighi O. *In Silico* study of the structure and ligand preference of pyruvate kinases from *Cyanobacterium synechocystis* sp. PCC 6803. Appl Biochem Biotechnol 2021; 193(11): 3651-71.
[http://dx.doi.org/10.1007/s12010-021-03630-9] [PMID: 34347252]

[27]   Behbahani M, Moradi M, Mohabatkar H. *In silico* design of a multi-epitope peptide construct as a potential vaccine candidate for Influenza A based on neuraminidase protein. *In Silico* Pharmacol 2021; 9(1): 36.
[http://dx.doi.org/10.1007/s40203-021-00095-w] [PMID: 33987075]

[28]   Joshi DM, Patel J, Bhatt H. *In silico* study to quantify the effect of exercise on surface GLUT4 translocation in diabetes management. Netw Model Anal Health Inform Bioinform 2021; 10(1): 1.
[http://dx.doi.org/10.1007/s13721-020-00274-3]

[29]   Joshi DM, Patel J, Bhatt H. *In silico* study to optimize the dosage of oleuropein with metformin in diabetes management Iraqi J Sci 2023.
[http://dx.doi.org/10.24996/ijs.2023.64.8.14]

[30]   Joshi DM, Patel J, Bhatt H. Dosage optimization of metformin and oleuropein along with exercise in diabetes management. In: AIP Conference Proceedings. 2023.
[http://dx.doi.org/10.1063/5.0149280]

[31]   Taldaev A, Terekhov R, Nikitin I, Zhevlakova A, Selivanova I. Insights into the pharmacological effects of flavonoids: The systematic review of computer modeling. Int J Mol Sci 2022; 23(11): 6023.
[http://dx.doi.org/10.3390/ijms23116023] [PMID: 35682702]

[32]   Visentin R, Cobelli C, Dalla Man C. A software interface for *in silico* testing of type 2 diabetes treatments. Comput Methods Programs Biomed 2022; 223: 106973.
[http://dx.doi.org/10.1016/j.cmpb.2022.106973] [PMID: 35792365]

[33]   Zainab B, Ayaz Z, Alwahibi MS, *et al. In-silico* elucidation of *Moringa oleifera* phytochemicals against *Diabetes mellitus*. Saudi J Biol Sci 2020; 27(9): 2299-307.
[http://dx.doi.org/10.1016/j.sjbs.2020.04.002] [PMID: 32884411]

[34]   Timo GO, Reis RSSV, Melo AF, Costa TVL, Magalhães PO, Homem-de-Mello M. Predictive power of *in silico* approach to evaluate chemicals against m. tuberculosis: A systematic review. Pharmaceuticals (Basel) 2019; 12(3): 135.
[http://dx.doi.org/10.3390/ph12030135] [PMID: 31527425]

[35]   Siddaway AP, Wood AM, Hedges LV. How to do a systematic review: a best practice guide for conducting and reporting narrative reviews, meta-analyses, and meta-syntheses. Annu Rev Psychol 2019; 70(1): 747-70.
[http://dx.doi.org/10.1146/annurev-psych-010418-102803] [PMID: 30089228]

[36]   Pollock A, Berge E. How to do a systematic review. Int J Stroke 2018; 13(2): 138-56.
[http://dx.doi.org/10.1177/1747493017743796] [PMID: 29148960]

[37]   Sacan A, Ekins S, Kortagere S. Applications and limitations of *in silico* models in drug discovery. Methods Mol Biol 2012; 910: 87-124.
[http://dx.doi.org/10.1007/978-1-61779-965-5_6] [PMID: 22821594]

[38]   Gangrade D, Sawant G, Mehta A. Re-thinking drug discovery: *In silico* method. J Chem Pharm Res 8 Available from:www.jocpr.com

[39]   Ji Z, Yan K, Li W, *et al.* Mathematical and computational modeling in complex biological systems. BioMed Research International 2017.
[http://dx.doi.org/10.1155/2017/5958321]

CHAPTER 2

Foundations of Diabetes Technology

Abstract: This chapter covers the foundations of diabetes technology, discussing important topics like disease mechanisms, causes, risk factors, and associated complications. An urgent need for advancements in diabetes technology is emphasized so that it can reduce the complications associated with diabetes and enhance the lifestyle of affected individuals with preventive healthcare. It further discusses the classes of molecules and the genetic-level analysis of drug-receptor interactions, along with the role of receptors and drugs in detail. The kinetics of insulin with receptors are investigated, ranging from short-acting to ultra-long-acting insulin. There is a thorough discussion of *in silico* modeling, the effects of genetic variants on drug-receptor interactions, and the main medications used to treat diabetes. The chapter concludes with a discussion of the different risk factors and how they affect the management of diabetes. As a result, this chapter provides a solid research basis for both the present and upcoming areas of diabetes technology.

Keywords: Computational, Complications, Disease mechanism, Drug-receptor, *In silico*, Risk factors.

INTRODUCTION

Diabetes mellitus is a disease that has a negative impact on the metabolic function of the body, affecting millions of people all over the world. This condition causes severe health complications and lowers the quality of life. The number of people diagnosed with diabetes is increasing, and so is the need for efficient management and new technological solutions. Diabetes technology includes a variety of instruments, devices, and therapeutics aimed at better disease control and prevention of complications. This chapter delves into key concepts regulating diabetes technology, examining disease pathology, etiology, risk factors, and complications.

This chapter stresses the need to innovate diabetes technology to ameliorate the issues arising from the disease. It emphasizes how new techniques and computational models can disrupt the management and treatment of diabetes through personalized medicine. Among other important concepts are the mechanisms of action of insulin, insulin kinetics of the various types of insulin,

Darshna M. Joshi, Hardik Bhatt & Himanshu K. Patel

and the genomic pharmacodynamics of drug-receptor interactions. Furthermore, the chapter examines the precision of disease progression modeling and its uses in treatment and early intervention of risk factors.

There is no doubt that combining the newest technologies with medicine will add value and provide a better life for people living with diabetes. This chapter provides an understanding of foundational diabetes technology principles, as well as allows for realizing its transformative impact in the battle against the disease.

DISEASE MECHANISMS, COMPLICATIONS, AND SIGNALING PATHWAYS

According to the World Health Organization (WHO), diabetes mellitus is one of the fastest-growing chronic metabolic disorders in the world caused by the development of insulin resistance (Type 2 Diabetes Mellitus (T2DM)) or the failure of the body's pancreas to produce enough insulin (Type 1 Diabetes Mellitus (T1DM)). Diabetes is a condition characterized by impaired regulation of blood glucose levels due to dysfunction in insulin production or response. It is highly responsible for various comorbidities, including cardiovascular diseases, liver diseases, and major organ failure. Currently, 537 million people in the world are living with diabetes, and it is predicted to reach 783 million by 2045, as per the International Diabetes Federation (IDF) report [1 - 5]. Insulin resistance leads to unresponsive behaviors of the tissues to use glucose, and hence an imbalance in glucose occurs in the body that develops T2DM. The main factors that are responsible for the insulin resistance are unhealthy food habits, obesity, and no workouts [6 - 14, 14 - 19]. Diabetes is a chronic metabolic syndrome with no cure to date, thus increasing the risk of insulin resistance, obesity, cardiovascular diseases, and much more. The risk factors associated with the metabolic syndrome are shown in Fig.(**1**).

An alarming rise is observed in the global diabetes cases in comparison to 1990 [20]. The number has doubled from 7% to 14%, as per the world diabetes reports [21]. It is one of the fastest-growing metabolic disorders in the world that needs urgent attention [22]. The global healthcare cost associated with diabetes was 966 billion dollars in 2021 and is expected to rise to 1054 billion dollars in 2045, as per IDF reports [20]. As per the WHO report, to deal with this alarming rise, a 4th High-level Meeting of the United Nations General Assembly was held for the prevention and control of metabolic diseases like diabetes in September 2025. The agenda of the meeting was to address the root cause of diseases and discuss awareness and control treatments that can be applied to mitigate the disorder worldwide. Through this, the goal of 2050 to halt the diabetes epidemic is given utmost importance.

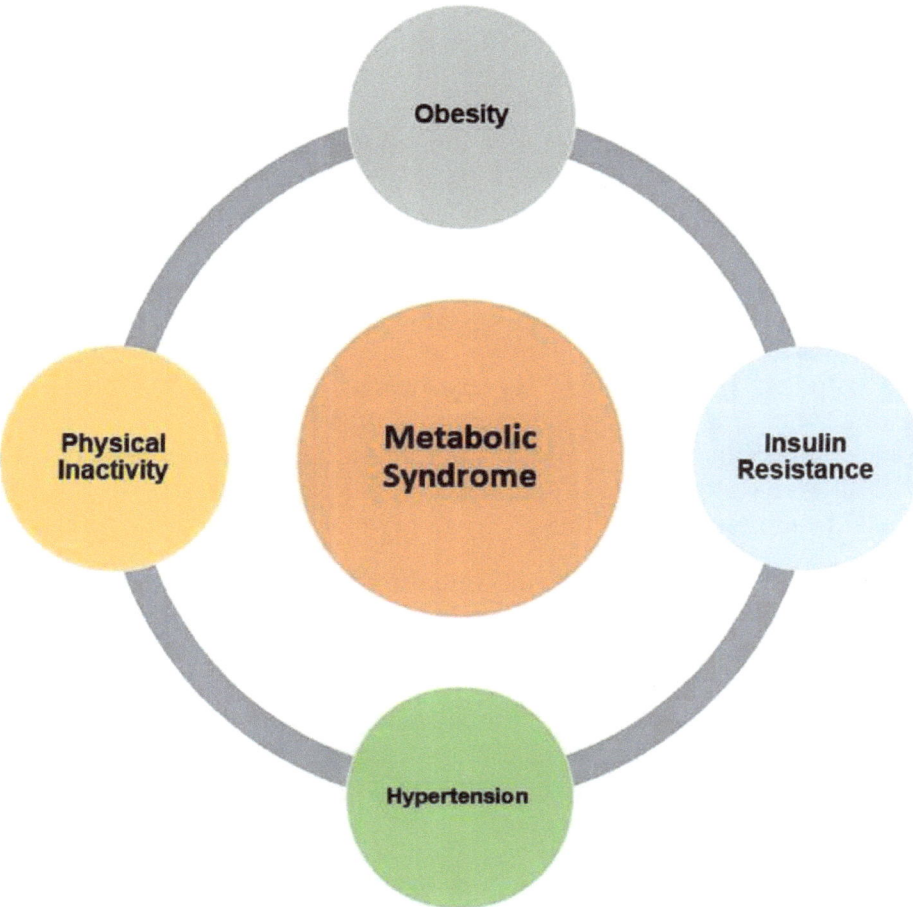

Fig. (1). Metabolic syndrome.

The complications associated with diabetes are not limited to vision problems, foot ulcers, kidney and liver diseases, cardiovascular issues, skin damage, and much more. People with diabetes are more prone to infections from their surroundings due to a weakened immune system. Ketoacidosis is another dangerous complication that needs urgent transfer of patients to the hospital. The person suffers from breathing issues as well as dehydration. Although it is a reversible condition, it requires urgent care [23 - 29].

Hypoglycemia is another condition of diabetes where the blood sugar levels are reduced drastically, leading to mortality. The signs are blurred vision, sweating, intense hunger, and absentmindedness. Similarly, hyperglycemia is a condition of an extreme rise in sugar levels. This is the most common condition affecting diabetic patients. It can be handled with a proper, balanced diet and exercise [27]. Diabetes is one such condition that adversely affects a person's organs. Macroangiopathy is a serious heart and vascular condition that causes hypertension and strokes. Diabetic retinopathy causes serious deterioration of vision due to damage to the eye vessels. Diabetic nephropathy results in renal insufficiency, while diabetic neuropathy causes muscle atrophy and difficulty in walking. Diabetic foot is another complication that causes wounds and ulcers, and vulnerability to infections with liver damage are the major complications associated with diabetes mellitus [27 - 29]. Thus, high blood pressure, stroke, cardiovascular diseases, and similar diseases are the major complications faced by diabetic patients. Hyperosmolar Hyperglycemic State (HHS) is another life-threatening emergency that only occurs with type 2 diabetes, causing very high blood sugar levels and leading to death if not treated on an urgent basis. All these complications rise even more if people with diabetes are not following a healthy lifestyle and eating a healthy diet.

Further, it is important to explore the signaling pathways associated with T2DM to delve deeper into the complexities and to understand the underlying mechanisms of the metabolic disorder. The signaling pathways play a crucial role in the research and development of treatment, as they show the path of action for the treatment to be applied. An insulin signaling pathway is a series of chemical reactions in the body that allows insulin to regulate blood sugar levels by helping cells absorb glucose. In diabetes, disruptions in this pathway impair glucose uptake, leading to high blood sugar.

The body regulates glucose homeostasis through this insulin signaling pathway. Disruptions in the insulin signaling pathway lead to the onset of T2DM. Complete mechanisms involved in the insulin signaling are still an open area of research, but here, we have discussed Sedaghat *et al.*'s model of insulin signaling, which covers the major components involved in the transduction of insulin signaling [30]. Many papers have discussed insulin signaling pathways that help engulf glucose through glucose transporter 4 (GLUT4) in the plasma membrane [30 - 46].

Insulin signaling pathways consist of a simple linear cascade structure of receptor and effector, as per conventional research. At the same time, it has been found in recent years that it is much more complex, with interactions involved. The basic pathways involved in insulin signal transduction are shown in Fig.(**2**), developed with the help of PowerPoint.

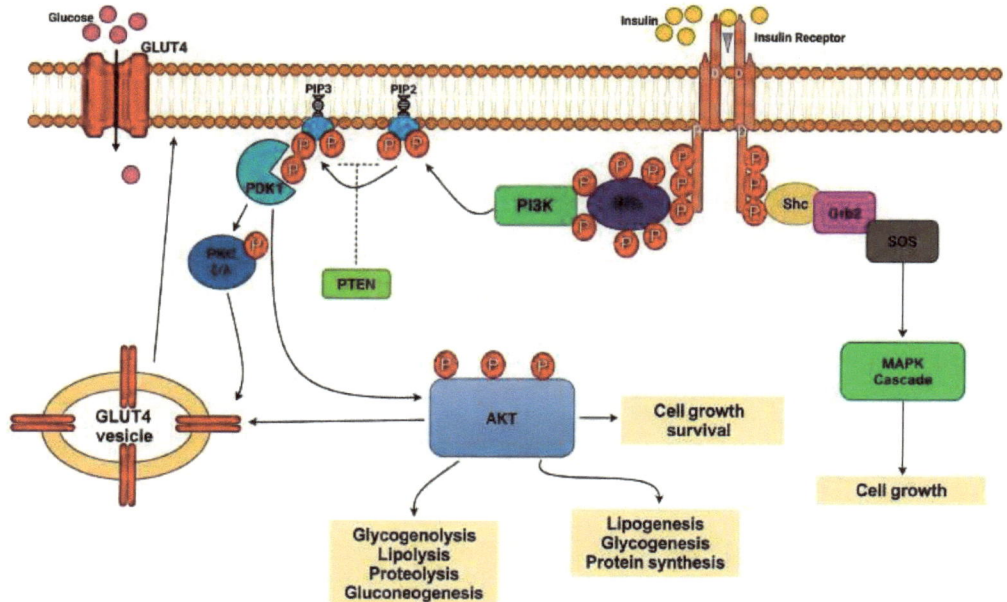

Fig. (2). Insulin signaling pathways.

In the beginning, insulin binds to the receptor available on the plasma membrane. As the binding occurs, auto-phosphorylation takes place, which leads to the activation of the insulin receptor. With this, insulin receptor substrate-1 (IRS1) gets phosphorylated and forms a complex with phosphatidylinositol-3-kinase (PI3K). With the catalyst IRS1-PI3K complex, phosphatidylinositol triphosphate (PIP3) is formed.

Phosphoinositide-dependent kinase 1 (PDK1) is used for allosteric interaction, which forms a complex PIP3-PDK1, resulting in the phosphorylation of protein kinases AKT and protein kinase C ζ (PKC ζ). With this activation, glucose transporter 4 (GLUT4) gets translocated to the plasma membrane through an unknown mechanism. As soon as GLUT4 is available on the plasma membrane, cells take up the glucose from the blood and thus maintain glucose homeostasis in the body. A number of other proteins and phosphates are involved in the pathways, like protein tyrosine phosphatase1B (PTP1B), PIP3 SHIP2, and PTEN (lipid phosphatases) [30, 47 - 54]. In T1DM, insulin production is severely reduced due to the loss of beta cells, impairing insulin signaling and glucose regulation.

Another pathway element that plays a major role in the GLUT4 translocation is the activation of Adenosine Monophosphate Kinase (AMPK) enzyme. Drugs like metformin, used for the treatment of T2DM, utilize this pathway to regulate glucose in the body. AMPK is a heterotrimeric complex. It is made up of catalytic α and regulatory β and γ subunits. When AMP binds to the γ subunit, the allosteric activation of the complex takes place. As a result, Thr172 gets phosphorylated, and this results in the regulation of glucose in the body. As AMPK is a cellular energy sensor, it is a crucial target for the treatment of T2DM [37, 55 - 76].

The testing and analysis of such complex insulin signal transduction pathways seem to be difficult, costly, and time-consuming tasks. Hence, it is proposed that *in silico* modeling can be performed, and various analyses can be easily carried out before opting for costly *in vivo* and *in vitro* analyses. This chapter thus further discusses the urgent need for advancements in diabetes technology.

THE URGENT NEED FOR ADVANCEMENTS IN DIABETES TECHNOLOGY

The growing global prevalence of diabetes has led to an urgency in the development of technologies that can help deal with the regulation of glucose. The current healthcare system is not able to cope with the tremendous rise in diabetes numbers. Although much development has taken place in terms of diabetes treatment, there is always a higher need for further innovations and research on glucose monitoring, insulin delivery, and glucose regulatory therapies that can help mitigate the condition. The world is working to eradicate the diabetes epidemic.

Advancement in diabetes technology is the need of the hour for millions of people in the world. Although there are multiple devices like Continuous Glucose Monitoring (CGM) systems, diabetes smart pens, insulin pumps, artificial pancreas systems, and more personalized treatment algorithms, it is essential that advancements and innovations take place to reduce the complications and provide a better quality of life for those living with diabetes. Moreover, in today's digital age, research on wearable devices, prediction-based health applications, remote monitoring, and other AI-based tools is very much needed to support the decision-making process for health practitioners [77 - 82].

Over the span of recent years, a radical transformation has been seen in diabetes management due to technological advancements. Major healthcare industries have shown interest in research and innovations in diabetes devices. Glucose monitoring is now possible on the fingertip, and management can take place easily through smartphones. Wearable devices like smartwatches with glucose meters and advanced technology monitor glucose levels every minute. With advancements in sensor technology, data analytics, and real-time management, it is possible to provide more seamless delivery of diabetes diagnostics and care.

Apart from invasive care, non-invasive glucose monitoring technologies, such as electromechanical, optical, and electrochemical, require evaluation these days. All these technologies should provide patient-friendly options to eliminate the need for the finger-prick test [79, 83 - 87].

More advanced technologies, such as Artificial Intelligence (AI) and Machine Learning (ML), can be used to provide personalized treatment. With this, predictions about the health of an individual can be made very easily through algorithms. These technologies can thus help provide precise treatments that improve outcomes and reduce risks. Patients can be empowered through health education and management tools, using various applications that provide guidance on nutrition, exercise, alternative therapy suggestions, and customized health plans with daily reminders. By this, each individual can receive personalized treatment with technological advancements and thus improve their diabetes condition, resulting in a reduction in long-term complications [86, 87].

Technological advancements are boosted with the help of *in silico* modeling, which uses computer simulations and computational models for analyzing the underlying mechanisms of various biological systems. With a detailed understanding of biological systems, advancements in diabetes technology play a crucial role. With the help of simulations, drug targets can be identified, genetic variations can be studied, and the effects of various types of disruptions can be studied and predicted. With *in silico* modeling, algorithms can be developed to predict insulin dose requirements well in advance based on past data analysis. The programming of an artificial pancreas can be possible with computational techniques. Also, various drug interactions can be studied with the help of computational models. Thus, with the ability to simulate various diabetes conditions and predict glucose levels, *in silico* modeling plays a critical role in the technological advancement of diabetes care [53, 88 - 97].

It uses computational methods of engineering to represent and analyze complex biological mechanisms. Various diseases are modeled, and predictions about the target therapies needed to solve complex biological phenomena are made using computational advancements [98, 99]. Advancements in computational methods have shown a proven improvement in the understanding of biological systems by healthcare researchers and computational scientists. As per the latest trends, advanced computational methods like Artificial Intelligence (AI)-based machine learning have successfully demonstrated predictions about sensitive targets for drug therapy as well as early detection of diseases, which can help manage the biological issues worldwide [98 - 104].

RECEPTORS, CONFIGURATION, AND SIGNIFICANCE: *IN SILICO* MODELING

Proteins that interact with various signaling molecules, like ligands and drugs, for the successful regulation of complex biological processes are known as receptors. For therapeutic interventions in diabetes, the receptors that play crucial roles are always targeted by researchers. Dysfunction of these receptors leads to the onset of both Type 1 and Type 2 diabetes. For drug discovery, the use of computational modeling techniques to model various interactions, configurations, and functions of receptors to better understand the underlying mechanism of diabetes is essential [95 - 97, 105 - 111]. With the help of *in silico* modeling, structural changes associated with mutations and conformational changes in the receptors are obtained, and this allows healthcare providers to identify crucial drug targets for enhancing glucose uptake *via* treatment of the downstream signaling pathways.

Below are the details about the receptors associated with diabetes, the role *in silico* modeling plays a significant role in the process, and their configurations.

Insulin Receptor (IR): The insulin receptor is a tyrosine kinase. It regulates glucose uptake, protein synthesis, and metabolism of lipids in the body. As explained in the signaling pathways section above, when the insulin binds to the insulin receptor, it becomes autophosphorylated and triggers the downstream signaling pathway *via* the PI3K-Akt pathway, thereby maintaining glucose and other anabolic processes. When this channel is disrupted, insulin resistance develops, resulting in the elevation of glucose levels [112 - 121].

- **Molecular Docking:** The binding of insulin to its receptors and how the insulin interacts at the active site are examined in docking studies. With the help of such simulations, binding energy at the site can be analyzed, and based on binding affinity, predictions about the future can be made if there is the presence of insulin resistance.
- **Molecular Dynamics (MD) Simulations:** To analyze the conformational flexibility of receptors and their dynamic response to insulin binding, MD simulations are used. The structural changes and shape changes of the insulin receptors can be observed, and the potential areas where insulin resistance has developed can be identified.
- **Homology Modeling:** When there is a limit on the experimental data and the structures of the receptors are unknown, homology modeling helps predict 3D structures based on known sequences and related protein structures. This enhances the study of unknown mechanisms involved in signal transduction.

Glucagon Receptor (GCGR): The regulation of glucose in the liver is done by the glucagon receptor (GCGR). Elevated glucose levels in the liver promote hepatic glucose production in both Type 1 and Type 2 diabetes mellitus, resulting in the development of hyperglycemia [122 - 125].

- **Docking and Virtual Screening:** The simulation for the analysis of how glucagon binds to the GCGR is performed through docking studies. With the help of this, one can identify the antagonists to block the activation of receptors, potentially reducing the production of excessive glucose in the liver. Additionally, virtual screening helps explore the large number of compound libraries to identify novel GCGR inhibitors.
- **Conformational Analysis:** The structural changes associated with GCGR upon ligand binding can be studied using MD simulations. With this, one can identify the underlying mechanisms linked with receptor mutations and uncontrolled glucagon secretion.
- **Binding Site Prediction:** To identify the effects of drugs on the binding site, computational methods are used. The modulation of the receptor's function can take place when a small molecule binds to the receptor, which results in the new therapeutic avenues.

GLP-1 Receptor (GLP-1R): Glucose homeostasis is maintained by the GLP-1 receptor. It is done so by enhancing the secretion of insulin, delaying the emptying of the stomach, as well as by inhibiting the release of glucagon. The agonists of the **GLP-1 receptor** are used to treat T2DM [107, 126 - 130].

- **Molecular Docking and Dynamics Simulations:** The optimal binding sites of GLP-1R can be identified using molecular docking. The analysis of conformational changes upon the binding of ligand helps in designing more effective GLP-1 agonists, which leads to improvements in pharmacokinetics and stability.
- **Pharmacophore Modeling:** Pharmacophore modeling is a computational method that identifies the essential chemical features of a drug needed to interact with a specific receptor in the body. In diabetes, it helps design drugs that effectively bind to receptors to regulate blood sugar levels.
- This modeling provides the critical chemical features of the analogs of GLP-1. It will thus give information regarding the receptor binding and activation. New compounds could be designed based on this that can mimic the performance of GLP-1's effects on insulin secretion.
- **Ligand-Receptor Interaction Studies:** The non-covalent interactions between GLP-1R and various other agonists are being studied, which

will help in the design and development of more potent and accurate drugs for diabetes management.

SGLT2 (Sodium-Glucose Cotransporter 2): The reabsorption of glucose in the kidneys is mediated by SGLT2. There is a class of drugs like empagliflozin, which are SGLT2 inhibitors. They are responsible for the excretion of glucose *via* urine and managing T2DM [131 - 142].

- **Molecular Docking:** How well SGLT2 inhibitors bind to the active site for the blocking of glucose reabsorption is studied with the help of molecular docking. Molecular docking helps design an optimal structure of inhibitors to enhance selectivity as well as potency.
- **Binding Site Identification:** *In silico* modeling tools are helpful to predict the active binding site of SGLT2 inhibitors. It also provides the details of interactions between various inhibitors and amino acids present in the transporter to promote better design.
- **Pharmacophore Modeling and Virtual Screening:** Virtual screening helps in the identification of novel SGLT2 inhibitors, and *in silico* pharmacophore modeling helps in the identification of molecular features crucial for the inhibition of SGLT2.

PPAR-γ (Peroxisome Proliferator-Activated Receptor Gamma): The metabolism of lipids, differentiation of adipocytes, and the regulation of insulin sensitivity are taken care of by a nuclear receptor called PPAR-γ. Agonists, like thiazolidinediones, help in the regulation of glucose by reducing insulin resistance [143 - 148].

- **Molecular Docking and Dynamics Simulations:** Identification of new ligands is done using computational analysis through docking studies. It provides the result of interactions of PPAR-γ agonists with the receptor and the associated conformational changes that take place upon binding.
- **Pharmacophore Modeling:** New modulators of PPAR-γ are designed with the help of pharmacophore modeling. It is helpful in the identification of the critical features of ligand-receptor binding, which thus leads to better drug development with fewer side effects.

Leptin Receptor (LEPR): The regulation of energy balance, insulin sensitivity, and appetite is carried out with the help of the leptin receptor. Leptin resistance plays a major role in obesity and the development of insulin resistance in T2DM [149 - 154].

- **Molecular Docking and Dynamics:** Molecular docking is used to simulate the behavior of the binding of leptin as well as its analogs to the receptor available at the site, while the conformational change in the structure of the leptin while binding takes place is analyzed using MD simulations. These detailed simulations help us in the analysis of the development of insulin resistance and enhance the identification of potential drug targets to promote leptin sensitivity.
- **Receptor Modeling:** When there is an absence of experimental structures, homology modeling is used to predict the 3D structure of the leptin receptor and its interaction with other modulating agents.

Adiponectin Receptors (AdipoR1, AdipoR2): Improvement in insulin sensitivity and regulation of blood glucose is taken care of by adiponectin receptors. Low levels of adiponectin contribute to the development of insulin resistance and obesity in T2DM [155 - 167].

- **Molecular Docking and Dynamics Simulations:** The interactions of adiponectin with its receptors (AdipoR1, AdipoR2) are studied using docking studies. The simulations help identify and modify the design of the ligands through which one can activate the receptors and hence enhance insulin sensitivity.
- **Binding Affinity Studies:** *In silico* modeling-based studies are used to estimate the binding affinity of receptors and, thus, find out the potential compounds that could mimic the benefits of adiponectin receptors to improve insulin sensitivity.

GPR40 (Free Fatty Acid Receptor 1): In response to fatty acids, GPR40 is involved in the secretion of insulin and also plays a critical role in the enhancement of glucose-based insulin secretion [168 - 173].

- **Docking and Dynamics Simulations:** Identification of novel ligands and the response of the receptors to deal with these agonists can be studied using molecular docking and dynamics simulations.
- **Receptor Structure Prediction:** Computational modeling tools help in the prediction of the 3D structure of the receptor that enables the design of agonists.

In silico modeling acts as a powerful tool for the study of diabetes receptors, the conformational and structural changes, and their interactions with drug molecules, as well as for the identification of potential drug targets that are helpful in drug discovery. These tools and models contribute to the time and cost effectiveness of the solutions provided.

INTERACTIONS OF DRUGS WITH RECEPTORS: GENETIC LEVEL ANALYSIS

The effect of genetic variations on the interaction between drug and receptor plays a crucial role in diabetes. These interactions can impact metabolism, efficacy, and safety, as the genetic variations affect the way medicines are Absorbed, Distributed, Metabolized, and Excreted (ADME). For the treatment of diabetes, drugs usually bind to the receptors or enzymes that regulate the blood glucose levels. Genetic variations highly impact the binding affinity of drugs to the receptors. Diabetes is treated with nine major classes of drugs [174]. Pharmacologically, diabetes is treated with these nine major classes of approved drugs. Pharmacogenetics provides data that can help suggest personalized medicine for diabetes mellitus [174 - 182].

An article by Shalini Singh *et al.* shows the pharmacogenetic studies update in T2DM. Several classes of drugs and their associations with genetic variations related to diabetes are discussed in detail. α-Glucosidase inhibitors, dipeptidyl peptidase-4 (DPP-4) inhibitors, glucagon-like peptide-1 (GLP-1) agonists, biguanides, sulfonylureas, meglitinides, thiazolidinediones (TZDs), sodium-glucose co-transporter-2 inhibitors, insulin, and its analogs are several classes of drugs that are preferred for diabetes [174, 180, 183]. The primary tissue targets of major anti-diabetic drugs [184] are shown in Fig.(**3**).

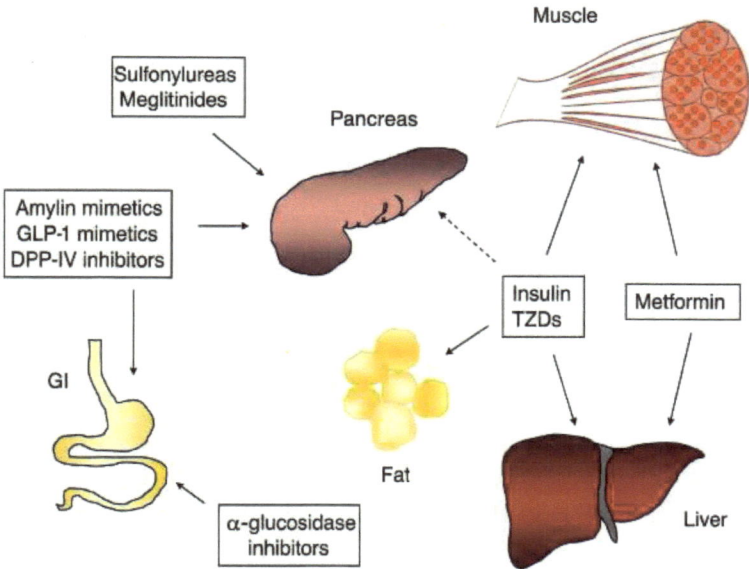

Fig. (3). Tissue targets of anti-diabetic drugs.

It is clearly observed that several classes of drugs have multi-organ effects. Each drug interacts with the relevant receptors and produces a glucose-reducing outcome to maintain metabolism in the body. The role of each class of drugs is shown in Table **1** [180].

Table 1. Various classes of drugs and genes involved in diabetes [180].

Class	Common medical representatives	Mechanism of action	Candidate genes involved in pharmacotherapy
Biguanide	Metformin	AMP-kinase activation	SLC22A1, SLC22A2, SLC22A3, SLC47A1, SLC47A2
Sulfonylureas	Gliburide, gliclazide, Glimepiride, glipizide	Inhibition of the KATP channel on the plasma membrane of ß-cells	KCNJ11, ABCC8, CYP2C9, TCF7L2
Thiazolidinediones	Pioglitazone, rosiglitazone	Activates PPAR-y	PPAR-y, ADIPOQ, TNF- CI, LEP, CYP2C8
Meglitinides	Nateglinide, repaglinide	Inhibition of the KATP channel on the plasma membrane of ß-cells	SLCOB1, CYP2C8, KCNQ1, SLC30A8, KCNJ11, TCF7L2
DPP-4 inhibitors	Alogliptin, linagliptin, saxagliptin, sitagliptin, vildagliptin	Inhibits DPP-4, Affect GLP-1 receptor pathway	Possibly TCF7L2
α-glucosidase inhibitors	Acarbose, miglitol, voglibose	Inhibits intestinal α-glucosidase	Yet to identify?
SGLT-2 inhibitors	Canagliflozin, dapagliflozin, empagliflozin	Inhibits SGLT2 transporters in the kidney	Yet to identify?
GLP-1 agonist	Exenatide, liraglutide	Activate GLP-1 receptor	Yet to identify?

α-Glucosidase Inhibitors

α-Glucosidase inhibitors like acarbose and miglitol work in the small intestine by inhibiting the enzyme α-glucosidase. As a result of this, the breakdown of complex carbohydrates into glucose is prevented, and this leads to the reduction of postprandial blood glucose levels. When genetic variations take place in the Glucocorticoid Receptor (GR), it may impact the efficacy of the drugs. One such example is the variation in the ABCB1 gene, which affects drug absorption [185 - 190].

Dipeptidyl Peptidase-4 (DPP-4) Inhibitors

DPP-4 inhibitors like sitagliptin and saxagliptin help block the enzyme DPP-4. This results in the inactivation of hormones like GLP-1. As a result, an enhancement in GLP-1 activity takes place. This promotes the production of insulin for meals and the inhibition of glucagon release, which results in the reduction of blood glucose levels. Genetic variations in DPP-4 may influence the metabolic effects and thus result in changes in therapeutic targets [191 - 197].

Glucagon-Like Peptide-1 (GLP-1) Agonists

GLP-1 agonists like liraglutide, semaglutide, and exenatide are mimetics of the natural hormone GLP-1, which stimulates the secretion of insulin in a glucose-dependent manner. As a result, glucagon secretion gets inhibited while promoting overfilling and reducing the emptying of the stomach. Any sort of genetic variations in GLP-1 influence drug efficacy [198 - 203].

Biguanides (*E.g.*, Metformin)

The production of glucose in the liver is inhibited primarily by biguanides, like metformin, which is the first-line treatment for type 2 diabetes. This leads to the improvement in insulin sensitivity and promotion of glucose uptake in muscle cells. The effectiveness and efficacy of metformin are impacted by the genetic variations in the AMPK. As metformin causes AMPK to get activated and hence maintain blood glucose, genetic variations cause the signals to get interrupted and thus reduce glucose uptake. Also, MTRR genetic variation influences the gastrointestinal issues that are involved in the metabolism of vitamin B12 [204 - 207].

Sulfonylureas

The binding of sulfonylurea receptor (SUR1) to sulfonylureas like glibenclamide and glimepiride leads to the closure of the potassium channel. This causes depolarization of the plasma membrane and secretion of insulin. Genetic variations in the KCNJ11 gene, which is responsible for encoding Kir6.2 (a subunit of the K_ATP channel), can affect the response to sulfonylureas. Mutations in KCNJ11 may lead to the reduction of the drug's ability to stimulate the secretion of insulin. Genetic variations in CYP2C9 also impact the clearance of drugs [208 - 211].

Meglitinides

Meglitinides like repaglinide and nateglinide stimulate the release of insulin from the pancreas because of binding to the potassium channel. Just like sulfonylureas, genetic variations influence the response to meglitinides and the metabolism of drugs for glucose reduction [212 - 217].

Thiazolidinediones (TZDs)

Thiazolidinediones like pioglitazone and rosiglitazone are PPAR-γ (peroxisome proliferator-activated receptor gamma) agonists. They are responsible for the improvement of insulin sensitivity in the peripheral tissues, such as muscle, liver, and adipose tissue. Genetic variations in the PPARG gene can alter the patient's response to TZDs and impact the receptor activity for glucose reduction [218 - 224].

Sodium-Glucose Co-Transporter-2 (SGLT2) Inhibitors

The blockage of SGLT2 transporters in the kidneys is done with the help of inhibitors like dapagliflozin and canagliflozin. As a result, the reabsorption of glucose is reduced, and it thus enhances glucose excretion in urine. Genetic variations in the SLC5A2 gene may have a crucial impact on this transporter, which alters the reabsorption rates and hence affects the glucose levels in diabetes [225 - 231].

Insulin and its Analogs

Insulin and its analogues, like insulin aspart, insulin glargine, and insulin lispro, are hormones that enhance glucose uptake in muscle, adipose tissues, and liver to maintain glucose homeostasis. The genetic variations in insulin receptors may have an impact on the target cells to the insulin, which imbalances the glucose control in the body. Insulin and its analogs have variation in the effectiveness over the binding and uptake signaling pathways for glucose homeostasis [232 - 238].

INSULIN KINETICS: DETAILED DISCUSSION ON DIVERSE CLASSES OF MOLECULES

Insulin is a hormone that is essential for energy regulation and hence maintains blood glucose levels. The kinetics of insulin include absorption, distribution, metabolism, and excretion of the hormone. It plays a crucial role in the understanding of diabetes management and other therapeutic interventions. There are various classes of insulin molecules with different pharmacokinetic profiles that are affected by multiple factors and hence cause a critical impact on glucose regulation in the body with their kinetics [239, 240].

Variations in the onset, peak action, and duration are observed in the insulin molecules because of their molecular structure. These differences arise due to the modification by various amino acid substitutions [241]. On the basis of pharmacokinetic properties, there are mainly 5 classes of insulin, which are discussed in detail in Table **2** [242].

Table 2. Types of insulin and their duration [242].

Type of Insulin	How long it takes to start working	How long it lasts	Examples
Rapid-acting insulin	15 minutes	2 to 4 hours	Insulin aspart (Novolog) Insulin lispro (Humalog) Insulin glulisine (Apidra)
Regular insulin	30 minutes	3 to 6 hours	Insulin regular (Novolin R)
Intermediate-acting insulin	1 to 2 hours	12 hours	NPH (Novolin N)
Long-acting insulin	2 to 4 hours	24 hours	Insulin detemir (Levemir) Insulin glargine (Lantus, Basaglar)
Ultra-long-acting insulin	6 hours	36 to 42 hours	Insulin degludec (Tresiba) Insulin glargine U300 (Toujeo)
Inhaled insulin	12–15 minutes	3 hours	Inhaled insulin (Afrezza)

Rapid-acting insulin is used to control and regulate postprandial glucose spikes in the body. The analogs of insulin are absorbed quickly, which leads to faster onset and thus enhances the physiological insulin response to the intake of food [243, 244]. Regular insulin or short-acting insulin has a slower absorption rate and hence a delay in the peak action is observed. This makes it suitable for pre-meal administration for controlling blood sugar postprandially. This is a more stable form, which is dissociated into monomers before absorption, and hence delays the onset in comparison to rapid-acting insulins [245 - 247]. Intermediate-acting insulin has slower absorption rates. It is due to the presence of protamine that forms a crystalline complex and hence delays dissociation and release of insulin [248].

Long-acting insulin provides a basal level of insulin for an extended period to control fasting glucose levels, which leads to slow absorption [248]. Ultra-lon--lasting insulin has even longer durations to act. It forms multi-hexamers and slowly dissociates, which makes it take longer for insulin to release in a steady form [249 - 251].

Several factors influence the action and pharmacokinetics of insulin, which include absorption, distribution, metabolism, and excretion. Absorption of insulin depends on the type of insulin used, the injection site, and the blood flow. Once the insulin is absorbed, it is distributed in the bloodstream based on the form of insulin, whether it is free or bound. After distribution, the metabolism of insulin takes place in the liver and kidneys with the help of degradation enzymes. Once it is metabolized, excretion takes place through the kidneys. The renal clearance depends largely on the patients' characteristics, like age, gender, weight, physical activity involved, food habits, stress, obesity, and use of diabetes technology for diabetes management [239, 240, 252].

RISK FACTORS IN DIABETES AND THEIR IMPLICATIONS

Diabetes is one of the widespread diseases in the world. It is not only caused by obesity, but a lack of healthy food habits and physical exercise may also lead to the onset of metabolic disorders. As per reports, in the USA, 90-95% of people with diabetes have inactive lifestyles. Among all the risk factors shown in Fig.(**4**), obesity is one of the major reasons responsible for diabetes.

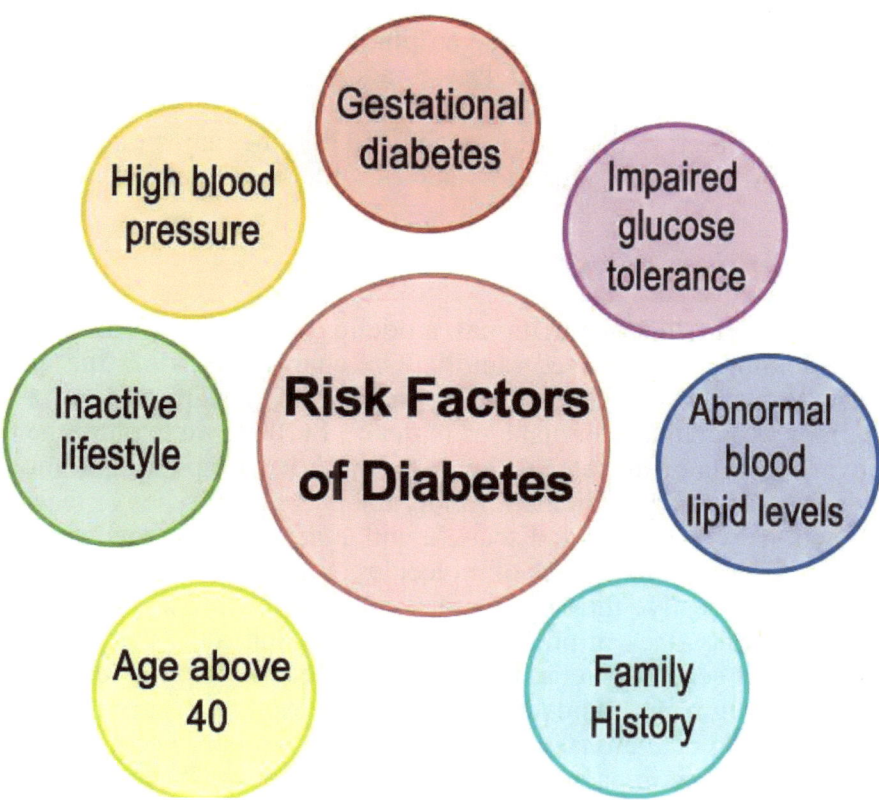

Fig. (4). Risk Factors for diabetes.

There are other factors related to family history and age. Gestational diabetes is another factor that enhances the risk of developing diabetes after pregnancy. Being overweight, frequent smoking habits, alcohol consumption, depression, and stress contribute to the onset of diabetes among individuals. Additionally, having irregular blood pressure can play a major role in developing diabetes. Also, some irreversible factors so far are family history due to genetics. People with diabetes in their family are at a higher risk of developing the same.

Leila Ismail *et al.* [253] have provided insights into the risk factors that are responsible for developing diabetes. They carried out a systematic literature survey by referring to reputed databases like Scopus, Springer, Web of Science, PubMed, and others. It is thereby recommended that early identification and preventive care with a healthy lifestyle and diet are the major ways that can help manage diabetes [254 - 257].

Yanling Wu *et al.* [258] discussed the risk factors that contribute to diabetes and the recent advancements that have taken place in the development of diabetes. They discussed various significant factors and their impact on the mechanism involved in diabetes. Also, statistical models associated with the prediction of diabetes were explored in detail. It is concluded that the major implication of the diabetes epidemic is the genetic factors and their interaction with the environment.

CONCLUDING REMARKS

With advancements in computational modeling and therapeutic innovations, diabetes technology has evolved rapidly. The chapter discusses the underlying mechanism of the insulin signaling pathways, insulin dynamics, and complications associated with diabetes in detail. Further, we explore the urgency in the advancements of diabetes technology and how computational models can help advise personalized medicine for individuals. Various types of receptors and their interactions with drugs are discussed with a genetic-level analysis. Also, the insulin kinetics for various classes of molecules are explored with the dynamics of types of insulin. Lastly, the risk factors concerned with the development of diabetes, like obesity, lack of physical activity, and unhealthy diet, are discussed. It is observed that genetic-level analysis with the help of *in silico* modeling, along with the underlying mechanisms involved in diabetes, holds a promising solution for early prediction of the onset of the metabolic disorder. These computational models can drastically impact the healthcare costs and time, and hence enhance the life of individuals with diabetes. As we move forward, interdisciplinary collaboration and innovation will be crucial in transforming diabetes management, offering new hope for millions worldwide.

CONSENT FOR PUBLICATION

We hereby give consent for publication.

REFERENCES

[1]   IDF International diabetes federation, the IDF consensus worldwide definition of the metabolic syndrome. Int Diabetes Fed. 2006; p. 24.

[2]   Dianna J Magliano *et al* IDF Diabetes Atlas 2022. Available from: https://diabetesatlas.org/idfawp/resource-files/2021/07/IDF_Atlas_10th_Edition_2021.pdf

[3]   - . The IDF consensus worldwide definition of the metabolic syndrome. Obes Metab 2005; 2(3): 47-9.
[http://dx.doi.org/10.14341/2071-8713-4854]

[4]   International Diabetes Federation. The IDF consensus worldwide definition of the metabolic syndrome. International Diabetes Federation 2005; 2010: 24.

[5]   Internation Diabetes Federation IDF Diabetes Atlas. 9th ed., International Diabetes Federation 2019.

[6]   Samuel VT, Shulman GI. The pathogenesis of insulin resistance: Integrating signaling pathways and substrate flux. J Clin Invest 2016; 126(1): 12-22.
[http://dx.doi.org/10.1172/JCI77812] [PMID: 26727229]

[7]   Kahn SE, Cooper ME, Del Prato S. Pathophysiology and treatment of type 2 diabetes: Perspectives on the past, present, and future. Lancet 2014; 383(9922): 1068-83.
[http://dx.doi.org/10.1016/S0140-6736(13)62154-6] [PMID: 24315620]

[8]   Zaccardi F, Webb DR, Yates T, *et al.* Pathophysiology of type 1 and type 2 diabetes mellitus: A 90-year perspective. Postgraduate Medical Journal; 92. Epub ahead of print 2016.
[http://dx.doi.org/10.1136/postgradmedj-2015-133281]

[9]   Petersen MC, Shulman GI. Mechanisms of insulin action and insulin resistance. Physiol Rev 2018; 98(4): 2133-223.
[http://dx.doi.org/10.1152/physrev.00063.2017] [PMID: 30067154]

[10]   DeFronzo RA, Ferrannini E, Groop L, *et al.* Type 2 diabetes mellitus. Nat Rev Dis Primers 2015; 1(1): 15019.
[http://dx.doi.org/10.1038/nrdp.2015.19] [PMID: 27189025]

[11]   Olokoba AB, Obateru OA, Olokoba LB. Type 2 diabetes mellitus: A review of current trends. Oman Med J 2012; 27(4): 269-73.
[http://dx.doi.org/10.5001/omj.2012.68] [PMID: 23071876]

[12]   Dunger DB, Ahmed ML. Diabetes In: Growth Disorders, Second Edition. 2007.
[http://dx.doi.org/10.7748/ns.31.19.64.s46]

[13]   Ozougwu O. The pathogenesis and pathophysiology of type 1 and type 2 diabetes mellitus. J Physiol Pathophysiol 2013; 4(4): 46-57.
[http://dx.doi.org/10.5897/JPAP2013.0001]

[14]   DeFronzo RA. Pathogenesis of type 2 diabetes mellitus. Med Clin North Am 2004; 88(4): 787-835, ix.
[http://dx.doi.org/10.1016/j.mcna.2004.04.013] [PMID: 15308380]

[15]   Kaul KL. Preparing pathology for precision medicine: challenges and opportunities. Virchows Arch 2017; 471(2): 141-6.
[http://dx.doi.org/10.1007/s00428-017-2141-z] [PMID: 28512674]

[16]   Rachek LI. *Glucose Homeostatis and the Pathogenesis of Diabetes Mellitus.* 2014.
[http://dx.doi.org/10.1016/B978-0-12-800101-1.00008-9]

[17]   Stumvoll M, Goldstein BJ, van Haeften TW. Type 2 diabetes: principles of pathogenesis and therapy. Lancet. 2005 Apr 9-15;365(9467):1333–46. doi: 10.1016/S0140-6736(05)61032-X. PMID: 15823385.

[18]   Zaccardi F, Webb DR, Yates T, *et al.* Pathophysiology of type 1 and type 2 diabetes mellitus: A 90-year perspective. *Postgraduate Medical Journal*; 92. Epub ahead of print 2016.
[http://dx.doi.org/10.1136/postgradmedj-2015-133281]

[19] Donath MY, Shoelson SE. Type 2 diabetes as an inflammatory disease. Nat Rev Immunol 2011; 11(2): 98-107.
[http://dx.doi.org/10.1038/nri2925] [PMID: 21233852]

[20] Sun H, Saeedi P, Karuranga S, *et al.* IDF Diabetes Atlas: Global, regional and country-level diabetes prevalence estimates for 2021 and projections for 2045. Diabetes Res Clin Pract 2022; 183: 109119.
[http://dx.doi.org/10.1016/j.diabres.2021.109119] [PMID: 34879977]

[21] Diabetes: A defining disease of the 21st century. Lancet 2023; 401(10394): 2087.
[http://dx.doi.org/10.1016/S0140-6736(23)01296-5]

[22] Hossain MJ, Al-Mamun M, Islam MR. Diabetes mellitus, the fastest growing global public health concern: Early detection should be focused. Health Sci Rep 2024; 7(3): e2004.
[http://dx.doi.org/10.1002/hsr2.2004] [PMID: 38524769]

[23] Silva EFF, Ferreira CMM, De Pinho L. Risk factors and complications in type 2 diabetes outpatients. Rev Assoc Med Bras63 2017.

[24] Nathan DM. Long-term complications of diabetes mellitus. N Engl J Med 1993; 328(23): 1676-85.
[http://dx.doi.org/10.1056/NEJM199306103282306] [PMID: 8487827]

[25] Shojima N, Yamauchi T. Progress in genetics of type 2 diabetes and diabetic complications. J Diabetes Investig 2023; 14(4): 503-15.
[http://dx.doi.org/10.1111/jdi.13970] [PMID: 36639962]

[26] Alberti KG, Zimmet PZ. Definition, diagnosis and classification of diabetes mellitus and its complications. Part 1: diagnosis and classification of diabetes mellitus provisional report of a WHO consultation. Diabet Med. 1998 Jul;15(7):539–53. doi: 10.1002/(SICI)1096-9136(199807)15:7 539::AID-DIA668 3.0.CO;2-S. PMID: 9686693.

[27] Elvira R, Urgilés M, Alexandra J, Pastuña T, González E, Lilia A, Romero-Sacoto LA, Ramírez Coronel A. Type 2 diabetes mellitus and chronic complications. 2020.

[28] Faselis C, Katsimardou A, Imprialos K, Deligkaris P, Kallistratos M, Dimitriadis K. Microvascular complications of type 2 diabetes mellitus. Curr Vasc Pharmacol 2020; 18(2): 117-24.
[http://dx.doi.org/10.2174/1570161117666190502103733] [PMID: 31057114]

[29] Reinehr T. Pathophysiology and complications of type 2 diabetes mellitus. Monatsschr Kinderheilkd 2005; 153(10): 927-35.
[http://dx.doi.org/10.1007/s00112-005-1224-0]

[30] Sedaghat AR, Sherman A, Quon MJ. A mathematical model of metabolic insulin signaling pathways. Am J Physiol Endocrinol Metab 2002; 283(5): E1084-101.
[http://dx.doi.org/10.1152/ajpendo.00571.2001] [PMID: 12376338]

[31] Joshi T, Singh AK, Haratipour P, *et al.* Targeting AMPK signaling pathway by natural products for treatment of diabetes mellitus and its complications. J Cell Physiol 2019; 234(10): 17212-31.
[http://dx.doi.org/10.1002/jcp.28528] [PMID: 30916407]

[32] Bergqvist N, Nyman E, Cedersund G, Stenkula KG. A systems biology analysis connects insulin receptor signaling with glucose transporter translocation in rat adipocytes. J Biol Chem 2017; 292(27): 11206-17.
[http://dx.doi.org/10.1074/jbc.M117.787515] [PMID: 28495883]

[33] Brännmark C, Nyman E, Fagerholm S, *et al.* Insulin signaling in type 2 diabetes: Experimental and modeling analyses reveal mechanisms of insulin resistance in human adipocytes. J Biol Chem 2013; 288(14): 9867-80.
[http://dx.doi.org/10.1074/jbc.M112.432062] [PMID: 23400783]

[34] White MF. Insulin signaling in health and disease. Science 2003; 302(5651): 1710-1.
[http://dx.doi.org/10.1126/science.1092952] [PMID: 14657487]

[35] Röckl KSC, Witczak CA, Goodyear LJ. Signaling mechanisms in skeletal muscle: Acute responses

and chronic adaptations to exercise. IUBMB Life 2008; 60(3): 145-53.
[http://dx.doi.org/10.1002/iub.21] [PMID: 18380005]

[36]   Turban S, Stretton C, Drouin O, *et al.* Defining the contribution of AMP-activated protein kinase (AMPK) and protein kinase C (PKC) in regulation of glucose uptake by metformin in skeletal muscle cells. J Biol Chem 2012; 287(24): 20088-99.
[http://dx.doi.org/10.1074/jbc.M111.330746] [PMID: 22511782]

[37]   M Lehnen A. Changes in the GLUT4 Expression by Acute Exercise, Exercise Training and Detraining in Experimental Models. J Diabetes Metab 2013; 1(S10)
[http://dx.doi.org/10.4172/2155-6156.S10-002]

[38]   Wu C, Jiang F, Wei K, Jiang Z. Exercise activates the PI3K-AKT signal pathway by decreasing the expression of 5α-reductase type 1 in PCOS rats. Sci Rep 2018; 8(1): 7982.
[http://dx.doi.org/10.1038/s41598-018-26210-0] [PMID: 29789599]

[39]   Carlon A. Modeling and Simulation of Insulin Signaling. University of Padova. 2013.

[40]   Zand H, Morshedzadeh N, Naghashian F. Signaling pathways linking inflammation to insulin resistance. Diabetes Metab Syndr 2017; 11 (Suppl. 1): S307-9.
[http://dx.doi.org/10.1016/j.dsx.2017.03.006] [PMID: 28365222]

[41]   Joshi DM, Patel J. A survey on control theoretic research paradigms of insulin signaling pathways study. In: Biotechnology and Biological Sciences-Proceedings of the 3rd International Conference of Biotechnology and Biological Sciences, BIOSPECTRUM. 85-91.
[http://dx.doi.org/10.1201/9781003001614-14]

[42]   Sulaimanov N, Klose M, Busch H, Boerries M. Understanding the MTOR signaling pathway *via* mathematical modeling. Wiley Interdiscip Rev Syst Biol Med 2017; 9(4): e1379.
[http://dx.doi.org/10.1002/wsbm.1379] [PMID: 28186392]

[43]   Kadowaki T, Ueki K, Yamauchi T, Kubota N. SnapShot: Insulin signaling pathways. Cell 2012; 148(3): 624-624.e1, 624.e1.
[http://dx.doi.org/10.1016/j.cell.2012.01.034] [PMID: 22304926]

[44]   Joshi DM, Darshna A, Joshi M, *et al. A Survey on Control Theoretic Research Paradigms of Insulin Signaling Pathways Study.*
[http://dx.doi.org/10.1201/9781003001614-14]

[45]   Charzyńska A, Nałęcz A, Rybiński M, Gambin A. Sensitivity analysis of mathematical models of signaling pathways. BioTechnologia 2012; 93(3): 291-308.
[http://dx.doi.org/10.5114/bta.2012.46584]

[46]   Chew YH, Shia YL, Lee CT, *et al.* Modeling of glucose regulation and insulin-signaling pathways. Mol Cell Endocrinol 2009; 303(1-2): 13-24.
[http://dx.doi.org/10.1016/j.mce.2009.01.018] [PMID: 19428987]

[47]   Di Camillo B, Carlon A, Eduati F, Toffolo GM. A rule-based model of insulin signalling pathway. BMC Syst Biol 2016; 10(1): 38.
[http://dx.doi.org/10.1186/s12918-016-0281-4] [PMID: 27245161]

[48]   Summer T. Sensitivity analysis in systems biology modelling and its application to a multi-scale model of blood glucose homeostasis 2010. Available from:http://eprints.ucl.ac.uk/19896/1/19896.pdf

[49]   Kwei E, Sanft K, Petzold L, *et al. Systems analysis of the insulin signaling pathway.* IFAC Epub ahead of prin 2008.
[http://dx.doi.org/10.3182/20080706-5-KR-1001.02686]

[50]   Vinod PK, Venkatesh KV. Quantification of signaling networks. J Indian Inst Sci 2008; 88: 1-26.

[51]   Joshi DM, Patel J, Bhatt H. *In silico* study to quantify the effect of exercise on surface GLUT4 translocation in diabetes management. Netw Model Anal Health Inform Bioinform 2021; 10(1): 1.
[http://dx.doi.org/10.1007/s13721-020-00274-3]

[52]   Joshi DM, Patel J. A survey on control theoretic research paradigms of insulin signaling pathways study. Biotechnol Biol Sci. 2019; pp. 85-91.
[http://dx.doi.org/10.1201/9781003001614-14]

[53]   Joshi D. Dynamic *in silico* model of type 2 diabetes treated with metformin combined with exercise: a Sobol sensitivity analysis. Avicenna J Pharm Res. 2022 Dec;3(2):91–97. doi: 10.34172/ajpr.1074.

[54]   Joshi DM, Patel J, Bhatt H. Robust adaptation of PKC ζ-IRS1 insulin signaling pathways through integral feedback control. Biomed Phys Eng Express 2021; 7(5): 055013.
[http://dx.doi.org/10.1088/2057-1976/ac182e] [PMID: 34315137]

[55]   Hardie DG, Sakamoto K. AMPK: A key sensor of fuel and energy status in skeletal muscle. Physiology (Bethesda) 2006; 21(1): 48-60.
[http://dx.doi.org/10.1152/physiol.00044.2005] [PMID: 16443822]

[56]   Cao S, Li B, Yi X, *et al.* Effects of exercise on AMPK signaling and downstream components to PI3K in rat with type 2 diabetes. PLoS One 2012; 7(12): e51709.
[http://dx.doi.org/10.1371/journal.pone.0051709] [PMID: 23272147]

[57]   Hardie DG, Hawley SA. AMP-activated protein kinase: the energy charge hypothesis revisited. BioEssays 2001; 23(12): 1112-9.
[http://dx.doi.org/10.1002/bies.10009] [PMID: 11746230]

[58]   Kurth-Kraczek EJ, Hirshman MF, Goodyear LJ, Winder WW. 5′ AMP-activated protein kinase activation causes GLUT4 translocation in skeletal muscle. Diabetes 1999; 48(8): 1667-71.
[http://dx.doi.org/10.2337/diabetes.48.8.1667] [PMID: 10426389]

[59]   Kjøbsted R, Wojtaszewski JFP, Treebak JT. Role of AMP-Activated Protein Kinase for Regulating Post-exercise Insulin Sensitivity. EXS 2016; 107: 81-126.
[http://dx.doi.org/10.1007/978-3-319-43589-3_5] [PMID: 27812978]

[60]   Bird SR, Hawley JA. Update on the effects of physical activity on insulin sensitivity in humans. BMJ Open Sport Exerc Med 2017; 2(1): e000143.
[http://dx.doi.org/10.1136/bmjsem-2016-000143] [PMID: 28879026]

[61]   Steinberg GR, Carling D. AMP-activated protein kinase: the current landscape for drug development. Nat Rev Drug Discov 2019; 18(7): 527-51.
[http://dx.doi.org/10.1038/s41573-019-0019-2] [PMID: 30867601]

[62]   Holmes B, Dohm GL. Regulation of GLUT4 gene expression during exercise. In: Medicine and Science in Sports and Exercise. 2004.
[http://dx.doi.org/10.1249/01.MSS.0000132385.34889.FE]

[63]   LaMoia TE, Shulman GI. Cellular and molecular mechanisms of metformin action. Endocr Rev 2021; 42(1): 77-96.
[http://dx.doi.org/10.1210/endrev/bnaa023] [PMID: 32897388]

[64]   Alkhateeb H, Al-Duais M, Qnais E. Beneficial effects of oleuropein on glucose uptake and on parameters relevant to the normal homeostatic mechanisms of glucose regulation in rat skeletal muscle. Phytother Res 2018; 32(4): 651-6.
[http://dx.doi.org/10.1002/ptr.6012] [PMID: 29356144]

[65]   Coccimiglio IF, Clarke DC. ADP is the dominant controller of AMP-activated protein kinase activity dynamics in skeletal muscle during exercise. PLOS Comput Biol 2020; 16(7): e1008079.
[http://dx.doi.org/10.1371/journal.pcbi.1008079] [PMID: 32730244]

[66]   Zhang Y, Wang Y, Bao C, *et al.* Metformin interacts with AMPK through binding to γ subunit. Mol Cell Biochem 2012; 368(1-2): 69-76.
[http://dx.doi.org/10.1007/s11010-012-1344-5] [PMID: 22644486]

[67]   Richter EA, Hargreaves M. Exercise, GLUT4, and skeletal muscle glucose uptake. Physiol Rev 2013; 93(3): 993-1017.

[http://dx.doi.org/10.1152/physrev.00038.2012] [PMID: 23899560]

[68]   Kristensen JM, Lillelund C, Kjøbsted R, *et al.* Metformin does not compromise energy status in human skeletal muscle at rest or during acute exercise: A randomised, crossover trial. Physiol Rep 2019; 7(23): e14307.
[http://dx.doi.org/10.14814/phy2.14307] [PMID: 31833226]

[69]   Hardie DG. AMP-activated protein kinase—an energy sensor that regulates all aspects of cell function. Genes Dev 2011; 25(18): 1895-908.
[http://dx.doi.org/10.1101/gad.17420111] [PMID: 21937710]

[70]   Miller RA, Chu Q, Le Lay J, *et al.* Adiponectin suppresses gluconeogenic gene expression in mouse hepatocytes independent of LKB1-AMPK signaling. J Clin Invest 2011; 121(6): 2518-28.
[http://dx.doi.org/10.1172/JCI45942] [PMID: 21606593]

[71]   Jiménez-Sánchez C, Olivares-Vicente M, Rodríguez-Pérez C, *et al.* AMPK modulatory activity of olive–tree leaves phenolic compounds: Bioassay-guided isolation on adipocyte model and *in silico* approach. PLoS One 2017; 12(3): e0173074.
[http://dx.doi.org/10.1371/journal.pone.0173074] [PMID: 28278224]

[72]   Gwinn DM, Shackelford DB, Egan DF, *et al.* AMPK phosphorylation of raptor mediates a metabolic checkpoint. Mol Cell 2008; 30(2): 214-26.
[http://dx.doi.org/10.1016/j.molcel.2008.03.003] [PMID: 18439900]

[73]   Sriwijitkamol A, Coletta DK, Wajcberg E, *et al.* Effect of acute exercise on AMPK signaling in skeletal muscle of subjects with type 2 diabetes: A time-course and dose-response study. Diabetes 2007; 56(3): 836-48.
[http://dx.doi.org/10.2337/db06-1119] [PMID: 17327455]

[74]   Wadley GD, Lee-Young RS, Canny BJ, *et al.* Effect of exercise intensity and hypoxia on skeletal muscle AMPK signaling and substrate metabolism in humans. Am J Physiol Endocrinol Metab 2006; 290(4): E694-702.
[http://dx.doi.org/10.1152/ajpendo.00464.2005] [PMID: 16263768]

[75]   Coughlan Rudy J valentine Neil B Ruderman Asish K Saha endocrinology KA, Saha AK. Diabetes, Metabolic Syndrome and Obesity: Targets and Therapy Dovepress AMPK activation: A therapeutic target for type 2 diabetes? Diabetes, Metab Syndr Obes Targets Ther 2014; 7-241.

[76]   Musi N, Fujii N, Hirshman MF, *et al.* AMP-activated protein kinase (AMPK) is activated in muscle of subjects with type 2 diabetes during exercise. Diabetes 2001; 50(5): 921-7.
[http://dx.doi.org/10.2337/diabetes.50.5.921] [PMID: 11334434]

[77]   Bode B, King A, Russell-Jones D, Billings LK. Leveraging advances in diabetes technologies in primary care: a narrative review. Ann Med 2021; 53(1): 805-16.
[http://dx.doi.org/10.1080/07853890.2021.1931427] [PMID: 34184589]

[78]   Zimmerman C, Albanese-O'Neill A, Haller MJ. Advances in type 1 diabetes technology over the last decade. Eur Endocrinol 2019; 15(2): 70-6.
[http://dx.doi.org/10.17925/EE.2019.15.2.70] [PMID: 31616496]

[79]   Boughton CK, Hovorka R. New closed-loop insulin systems. Diabetologia 2021; 64(5): 1007-15.
[http://dx.doi.org/10.1007/s00125-021-05391-w] [PMID: 33550442]

[80]   Bzowyckyj A. Updates and advances in technology for diabetes self-management. Pharmacy Today 2019; 25(5): 43-58.
[http://dx.doi.org/10.1016/j.ptdy.2019.04.024]

[81]   Beck RW, Bergenstal RM, Laffel LM, Pickup JC. Advances in technology for management of type 1 diabetes. Lancet 2019; 394(10205): 1265-73.
[http://dx.doi.org/10.1016/S0140-6736(19)31142-0] [PMID: 31533908]

[82]   Magni L, Raimondo DM, Bossi L, *et al.* Model predictive control of type 1 diabetes: An *in silico* trial. J Diabetes Sci Technol 2007; 1(6): 804-12.

[http://dx.doi.org/10.1177/193229680700100603] [PMID: 19885152]

[83]　Saha T, Del Caño R, Mahato K, *et al.* Wearable electrochemical glucose sensors in diabetes management: A comprehensive review. Chem Rev 2023; 123(12): 7854-89.
[http://dx.doi.org/10.1021/acs.chemrev.3c00078] [PMID: 37253224]

[84]　Heinemann L, Stuhr A. Self-measurement of blood glucose and continuous glucose monitoring - Is there only one future? In: European Endocrinology. 2018.
[http://dx.doi.org/10.17925/EE.2018.14.2.24]

[85]　Bailey L. Moving with technological advancements: Blood glucose monitoring from a district nurse's perspective. Br J Community Nurs 2022; 27(10): 480-4.
[http://dx.doi.org/10.12968/bjcn.2022.27.10.480] [PMID: 36194398]

[86]　Agarwal S, Simmonds I, Myers AK. The use of diabetes technology to address inequity in health outcomes: Limitations and opportunities. Curr Diab Rep 2022; 22(7): 275-81.
[http://dx.doi.org/10.1007/s11892-022-01470-3] [PMID: 35648277]

[87]　Akturk HK, Aloi J, Shah VN, *et al.* Recent advances in diabetes technology and activities of the american diabetes association diabetes technology interest group. Clin Diabetes 2024; 42(2): 316-21.
[http://dx.doi.org/10.2337/cd23-0080] [PMID: 38694248]

[88]　Visentin R, Cobelli C, Dalla Man C. A software interface for *in silico* testing of type 2 diabetes treatments. Comput Methods Programs Biomed 2022; 223: 106973.
[http://dx.doi.org/10.1016/j.cmpb.2022.106973] [PMID: 35792365]

[89]　Dieter C, Lemos NE, Corrêa NRF, Assmann TS, Crispim D. The impact of lncRNAs in diabetes mellitus: A systematic review and *in silico* analyses. Front Endocrinol (Lausanne) 2021; 12: 602597.
[http://dx.doi.org/10.3389/fendo.2021.602597] [PMID: 33815273]

[90]　Zainab B, Ayaz Z, Alwahibi MS, *et al.* In-silico elucidation of *Moringa oleifera* phytochemicals against diabetes mellitus. Saudi J Biol Sci 2020; 27(9): 2299-307.
[http://dx.doi.org/10.1016/j.sjbs.2020.04.002] [PMID: 32884411]

[91]　Gangrade D, Sawant G, Mehta A. Re-thinking drug discovery: *In silico* method Available from:www.jocpr.com

[92]　Brogi S, Ramalho TC, Kuca K, Medina-Franco JL, Valko M. Editorial: *In silico* methods for drug design and discovery. Front Chem 2020; 8: 612.
[http://dx.doi.org/10.3389/fchem.2020.00612] [PMID: 32850641]

[93]　Joshi DM, Patel J, Bhatt H. *In silico* study to optimize the dosage of oleuropein with metformin in diabetes management. Iraqi J Sci 2023.
[http://dx.doi.org/10.24996/ijs.2023.64.8.14]

[94]　Patek SD, Bequette BW, Breton M, *et al.* *In silico* preclinical trials: Methodology and engineering guide to closed-loop control in type 1 diabetes mellitus. J Diabetes Sci Technol 2009; 3(2): 269-82.
[http://dx.doi.org/10.1177/193229680900300207] [PMID: 20144358]

[95]　de Godoi RS, Almerão MP, da Silva FR. *In silico* evaluation of the antidiabetic activity of natural compounds from *Hovenia dulcis* Thunberg. J Herb Med 2021; 28: 100349.
[http://dx.doi.org/10.1016/j.hermed.2020.100349]

[96]　Medeiros I, Aguiar AJFC, Fortunato WM, *et al.* *In silico* structure-based design of peptides or proteins as therapeutic tools for obesity or diabetes mellitus: A protocol for systematic review and meta analysis. Medicine (Baltimore) 2023; 102(15): e33514.
[http://dx.doi.org/10.1097/MD.0000000000033514] [PMID: 37058011]

[97]　Gomes AFT, de Medeiros WF, de Oliveira GS, *et al.* *In silico* structure-based designers of therapeutic targets for diabetes mellitus or obesity: A protocol for systematic review. PLoS One 2022; 17(12): e0279039.
[http://dx.doi.org/10.1371/journal.pone.0279039] [PMID: 36508447]

[98]   Sleeman B, Jones P. Computational and mathematical methods in medicine. Comput Math Methods Med 2006; 7(1): 1-2.
[http://dx.doi.org/10.1080/10273660600818264] [PMID: 21812577]

[99]   Stead WW, Lin HS. *Computational technology for effective health care: Immediate steps and strategic directions.* 2009.
[http://dx.doi.org/10.17226/12572]

[100]   Qureshi R, Irfan M, Ali H, *et al.* Artificial intelligence and biosensors in healthcare and its clinical relevance: A review. IEEE Access 2023; 11: 61600-20.
[http://dx.doi.org/10.1109/ACCESS.2023.3285596]

[101]   Galizzi JP, Lockhart BP, Bril A. Applying systems biology in drug discovery and development. dmdi 2013; 28(2): 67-78.
[http://dx.doi.org/10.1515/dmdi-2013-0002] [PMID: 23612649]

[102]   Claus BL, Underwood DJ. Discovery informatics: its evolving role in drug discovery. Drug Discov Today 2002; 7(18): 957-66.
[http://dx.doi.org/10.1016/S1359-6446(02)02433-9] [PMID: 12546870]

[103]   Augen J. The evolving role of information technology in the drug discovery process. Drug Discov Today 2002; 7(5): 315-23.
[http://dx.doi.org/10.1016/S1359-6446(02)02173-6] [PMID: 11854055]

[104]   Choudhuri S, Yendluri M, Poddar S, *et al.* Recent advancements in computational drug design algorithms through machine learning and optimization. Kinases and Phosphatases 2023; 1(2): 117-40.
[http://dx.doi.org/10.3390/kinasesphosphatases1020008]

[105]   Mustafa HA, Albkrye AMS, AbdAlla BM, Khair MAM, Abdelwahid N, Elnasri HA. Computational determination of human *PPARG* gene: SNPs and prediction of their effect on protein functions of diabetic patients. Clin Transl Med 2020; 9(1): e7.
[http://dx.doi.org/10.1186/s40169-020-0258-1] [PMID: 32064572]

[106]   Escribano O, Beneit N, Rubio-Longás C, *et al.* The role of insulin receptor isoforms in diabetes and its metabolic and vascular complications. Journal of Diabetes Research 2017.
[http://dx.doi.org/10.1155/2017/1403206]

[107]   Hinnen D. Glucagon-like peptide 1 receptor agonists for type 2 diabetes. Diabetes Spectr 2017; 30(3): 202-10.
[http://dx.doi.org/10.2337/ds16-0026] [PMID: 28848315]

[108]   She M, Laudon M, Yin W. Melatonin receptors in diabetes: A potential new therapeutical target? Eur J Pharmacol 2014; 744: 220-3.
[http://dx.doi.org/10.1016/j.ejphar.2014.08.012] [PMID: 25160745]

[109]   Pan X, Tao S, Tong N. Potential therapeutic targeting neurotransmitter receptors in diabetes. Front Endocrinol (Lausanne) 2022; 13: 884549.
[http://dx.doi.org/10.3389/fendo.2022.884549] [PMID: 35669692]

[110]   Su J, Tang L, Luo Y, Xu J, Ouyang S. Research progress on drugs for diabetes based on insulin receptor/insulin receptor substrate. Biochem Pharmacol 2023; 217: 115830.
[http://dx.doi.org/10.1016/j.bcp.2023.115830] [PMID: 37748666]

[111]   Kokkinopoulou I, Diakoumi A, Moutsatsou P. Glucocorticoid receptor signaling in diabetes. Int J Mol Sci 2021; 22(20): 11173.
[http://dx.doi.org/10.3390/ijms222011173] [PMID: 34681832]

[112]   Mancusi C, Izzo R, di Gioia G, Losi MA, Barbato E, Morisco C. Insulin resistance the hinge between hypertension and type 2 diabetes. High Blood Press Cardiovasc Prev 2020; 27(6): 515-26.
[http://dx.doi.org/10.1007/s40292-020-00408-8] [PMID: 32964344]

[113]   Yaribeygi H, Farrokhi FR, Butler AE, Sahebkar A. Insulin resistance: Review of the underlying

molecular mechanisms. J Cell Physiol 2019; 234(6): 8152-61.
[http://dx.doi.org/10.1002/jcp.27603] [PMID: 30317615]

[114] Gavigan C, Donner T. Predictors of responsiveness to GLP-1 receptor agonists in insulin-treated patients with type 2 diabetes J Diabetes Res 2023.
[http://dx.doi.org/10.1155/2023/9972132]

[115] Reiter CEN, Wu X, Sandirasegarane L, *et al*. Diabetes reduces basal retinal insulin receptor signaling: Reversal with systemic and local insulin. Diabetes 2006; 55(4): 1148-56.
[http://dx.doi.org/10.2337/diabetes.55.04.06.db05-0744] [PMID: 16567541]

[116] Laakso M, Malkki M, Kekäläinen P, Kuusisto J, Deeb SS. Insulin receptor substrate-1 variants in non-insulin-dependent diabetes. J Clin Invest 1994; 94(3): 1141-6.
[http://dx.doi.org/10.1172/JCI117429] [PMID: 8083355]

[117] Tumminia A, Scalisi NM, Milluzzo A, Ettore G, Vigneri R, Sciacca L. Maternal diabetes impairs insulin and IGF-1 receptor expression and signaling in human placenta. Front Endocrinol (Lausanne) 2021; 12: 621680.
[http://dx.doi.org/10.3389/fendo.2021.621680] [PMID: 33776919]

[118] Kubota N, Kubota T, Kajiwara E, *et al*. Differential hepatic distribution of insulin receptor substrates causes selective insulin resistance in diabetes and obesity. Nat Commun 2016; 7(1): 12977.
[http://dx.doi.org/10.1038/ncomms12977] [PMID: 27708333]

[119] Fernández AM, Kim JK, Yakar S, *et al*. Functional inactivation of the IGF-I and insulin receptors in skeletal muscle causes type 2 diabetes. Genes Dev 2001; 15(15): 1926-34.
[http://dx.doi.org/10.1101/gad.908001] [PMID: 11485987]

[120] Lee YH, White MF. Insulin receptor substrate proteins and diabetes. Arch Pharm Res 2004; 27(4): 361-70.
[http://dx.doi.org/10.1007/BF02980074] [PMID: 15180298]

[121] Chen Y, Huang L, Qi X, Chen C. Insulin receptor trafficking: Consequences for insulin sensitivity and diabetes. Int J Mol Sci 2019; 20(20): 5007.
[http://dx.doi.org/10.3390/ijms20205007] [PMID: 31658625]

[122] Furió-Novejarque C, Sanz R, Ritschel TKS, *et al*. Modeling the effect of glucagon on endogenous glucose production in type 1 diabetes: On the role of glucagon receptor dynamics. Comput Biol Med 2023; 154: 106605.
[http://dx.doi.org/10.1016/j.compbiomed.2023.106605] [PMID: 36731362]

[123] Capozzi ME, D'Alessio DA, Campbell JE. The past, present, and future physiology and pharmacology of glucagon. Cell Metab 2022; 34(11): 1654-74.
[http://dx.doi.org/10.1016/j.cmet.2022.10.001] [PMID: 36323234]

[124] Cho YM, Merchant CE, Kieffer TJ. Targeting the glucagon receptor family for diabetes and obesity therapy. Pharmacol Ther 2012; 135(3): 247-78.
[http://dx.doi.org/10.1016/j.pharmthera.2012.05.009] [PMID: 22659620]

[125] Eriksson O, Velikyan I, Haack T, *et al*. Imaging of the glucagon receptor in subjects with type 2 diabetes. J Nucl Med 2021; 62(6): 833-8.
[http://dx.doi.org/10.2967/jnumed.118.213306] [PMID: 33097629]

[126] Bailey J, Coucha M, Bolduc DR, *et al*. GLP-1 receptor nitration contributes to loss of brain pericyte function in a mouse model of diabetes. Diabetologia 2022; 65(9): 1541-54.
[http://dx.doi.org/10.1007/s00125-022-05730-5] [PMID: 35687178]

[127] Wilbon SS, Kolonin MG. GLP1 receptor agonists—effects beyond obesity and diabetes. Cells 2023; 13(1): 65.
[http://dx.doi.org/10.3390/cells13010065] [PMID: 38201269]

[128] Chen X, Christensen AS, Knop FK, Vilsbøll T. Glucagon-like peptide 1 receptor agonists for the treatment of Type 2 diabetes. Ugeskr Laeger 2023; 181(12): 72.

[http://dx.doi.org/10.1117/12.2669050] [PMID: 30931886]

[129] García-Casares N, González-González G, de la Cruz-Cosme C, *et al.* Effects of GLP-1 receptor agonists on neurological complications of diabetes. Rev Endocr Metab Disord 2023; 24(4): 655-72.
[http://dx.doi.org/10.1007/s11154-023-09807-3] [PMID: 37231200]

[130] Nauck MA, Quast DR, Wefers J, Meier JJ. GLP-1 receptor agonists in the treatment of type 2 diabetes – state-of-the-art. Mol Metab 2021; 46: 101102.
[http://dx.doi.org/10.1016/j.molmet.2020.101102] [PMID: 33068776]

[131] Gadzhanova S, Pratt N, Roughead E. Use of SGLT2 inhibitors for diabetes and risk of infection: Analysis using general practice records from the NPS MedicineWise MedicineInsight program. Diabetes Res Clin Pract 2017; 130: 180-5.
[http://dx.doi.org/10.1016/j.diabres.2017.06.018] [PMID: 28646701]

[132] Danne T, Biester T, Kordonouri O. Combined SGLT1 and SGLT2 inhibitors and their role in diabetes care. Diabetes Technol Ther 2018; 20(S2): S2-69-, S2-77.
[http://dx.doi.org/10.1089/dia.2018.0081] [PMID: 29916741]

[133] Pinto LC, Rados DV, Remonti LR, Viana MV, Leitão CB, Gross JL. Dose-ranging effects of SGLT2 inhibitors in patients with type 2 diabetes: a systematic review and meta-analysis. Arch Endocrinol Metab 2022; 66(1): 68-76.
[http://dx.doi.org/10.20945/2359-3997000000440] [PMID: 35263050]

[134] Suzuki Y, Kaneko H, Okada A, *et al.* Comparison of cardiovascular outcomes between SGLT2 inhibitors in diabetes mellitus. Cardiovasc Diabetol 2022; 21(1): 67.
[http://dx.doi.org/10.1186/s12933-022-01508-6] [PMID: 35585590]

[135] Evans M, Hicks D, Patel D, Patel V, McEwan P, Dashora U. Optimising the benefits of SGLT2 inhibitors for type 1 diabetes. Diabetes Ther 2020; 11(1): 37-52.
[http://dx.doi.org/10.1007/s13300-019-00728-6] [PMID: 31813092]

[136] Chao EC, Henry RR. SGLT2 inhibition — A novel strategy for diabetes treatment. Nat Rev Drug Discov 2010; 9(7): 551-9.
[http://dx.doi.org/10.1038/nrd3180] [PMID: 20508640]

[137] Shaffner J, Chen B, Malhotra DK, Dworkin LD, Gong R. Therapeutic targeting of SGLT2: A new era in the treatment of diabetes and diabetic kidney disease. Front Endocrinol (Lausanne) 2021; 12: 749010.
[http://dx.doi.org/10.3389/fendo.2021.749010] [PMID: 34790170]

[138] Hropot T, Battelino T, Dovc K. Sodium-glucose co-transporter-2 inhibitors in type 1 diabetes: A scoping review. Horm Res Paediatr 2023; 96(6): 620-30.
[http://dx.doi.org/10.1159/000527653] [PMID: 36279850]

[139] Gomez-Peralta F, Abreu C, Lecube A, *et al.* Practical approach to initiating sglt2 inhibitors in type 2 diabetes. Diabetes Ther 2017; 8(5): 953-62.
[http://dx.doi.org/10.1007/s13300-017-0277-0] [PMID: 28721687]

[140] Vallon V. The mechanisms and therapeutic potential of SGLT2 inhibitors in diabetes mellitus. Annu Rev Med 2015; 66(1): 255-70.
[http://dx.doi.org/10.1146/annurev-med-051013-110046] [PMID: 25341005]

[141] Tang H, Dai Q, Shi W, Zhai S, Song Y, Han J. SGLT2 inhibitors and risk of cancer in type 2 diabetes: A systematic review and meta-analysis of randomised controlled trials. Diabetologia 2017; 60(10): 1862-72.
[http://dx.doi.org/10.1007/s00125-017-4370-8] [PMID: 28725912]

[142] Simes BC, MacGregor GG. Sodium-glucose cotransporter-2 (SGLT2) inhibitors: A clinician's guide. Diabetes Metab Syndr Obes 2019; 12: 2125-36.
[http://dx.doi.org/10.2147/DMSO.S212003] [PMID: 31686884]

[143] Janani C, Ranjitha Kumari BD. PPAR gamma gene – A review. Diabetes Metab Syndr 2015; 9(1): 46-

50.
[http://dx.doi.org/10.1016/j.dsx.2014.09.015] [PMID: 25450819]

[144]   Chandra A, Kaur P, Sahu SK, Mittal A. A new insight into the treatment of diabetes by means of pan PPAR agonists. Chem Biol Drug Des 2022; 100(6): 947-67.
[http://dx.doi.org/10.1111/cbdd.14020] [PMID: 34990085]

[145]   Blaschke F, Takata Y, Caglayan E, Law RE, Hsueh WA. Obesity, peroxisome proliferator-activated receptor, and atherosclerosis in type 2 diabetes. Arterioscler Thromb Vasc Biol 2006; 26(1): 28-40.
[http://dx.doi.org/10.1161/01.ATV.0000191663.12164.77] [PMID: 16239592]

[146]   Lecarpentier Y, Claes V, Vallée A, *et al.* Interactions between PPAR Gamma and the Canonical Wnt/Beta-Catenin Pathway in Type 2 Diabetes and Colon Cancer. PPAR Research 2017.
[http://dx.doi.org/10.1155/2017/5879090]

[147]   Zhong H, Geng R, Zhang Y, *et al.* Effects of peroxisome proliferator-activated receptor-gamma agonists on cognitive function: A systematic review and meta-analysis. Biomedicines 2023; 11(2): 246.
[http://dx.doi.org/10.3390/biomedicines11020246] [PMID: 36830783]

[148]   Ballav S, Biswas B, Sahu VK, Ranjan A, Basu S. PPAR-γ partial agonists in disease-fate decision with special reference to cancer. Cells 2022; 11(20): 3215.
[http://dx.doi.org/10.3390/cells11203215] [PMID: 36291082]

[149]   Gilloteaux J, Nicaise C, Sprimont L, Bissler J, Finkelstein JA, Payne WR. Leptin receptor defect with diabetes causes skeletal muscle atrophy in female obese Zucker rats where peculiar depots networked with mitochondrial damages. Ultrastruct Pathol 2021; 45(6): 346-75.
[http://dx.doi.org/10.1080/01913123.2021.1983099] [PMID: 34743665]

[150]   Olczyk P, Koprowski R, Komosinska-Vassev K, *et al.* Adiponectin, leptin, and leptin receptor in obese patients with type 2 diabetes treated with insulin detemir. Molecules 2017; 22(8): 1274.
[http://dx.doi.org/10.3390/molecules22081274] [PMID: 28758947]

[151]   Chen D, Xia G, Xu P, Dong M. Peripartum serum leptin and soluble leptin receptor levels in women with gestational diabetes. Acta Obstet Gynecol Scand 2010; 89(12): 1595-9.
[http://dx.doi.org/10.3109/00016349.2010.514040] [PMID: 20822472]

[152]   Adiga U, Banawalikar N, Mayur S, Bansal R, Ameera N, Rao S. Association of insulin resistance and leptin receptor gene polymorphism in type 2 diabetes mellitus. J Chin Med Assoc 2021; 84(4): 383-8.
[http://dx.doi.org/10.1097/JCMA.0000000000000507] [PMID: 33660621]

[153]   Wang B, Chandrasekera P, Pippin J. Leptin- and leptin receptor-deficient rodent models: Relevance for human type 2 diabetes. Curr Diabetes Rev 2014; 10(2): 131-45.
[http://dx.doi.org/10.2174/1573399810666140508121012] [PMID: 24809394]

[154]   Pereira S, O'Dwyer SM, Webber TD, *et al.* Metabolic effects of leptin receptor knockdown or reconstitution in adipose tissues. Sci Rep 2019; 9(1): 3307.
[http://dx.doi.org/10.1038/s41598-019-39498-3] [PMID: 30824713]

[155]   Peters KE, Beilby J, Cadby G, *et al.* A comprehensive investigation of variants in genes encoding adiponectin (ADIPOQ) and its receptors (ADIPOR1/R2), and their association with serum adiponectin, type 2 diabetes, insulin resistance and the metabolic syndrome. BMC Med Genet 2013; 14(1): 15.
[http://dx.doi.org/10.1186/1471-2350-14-15] [PMID: 23351195]

[156]   Sun X, Han R, Wang Z, Chen Y. Regulation of adiponectin receptors in hepatocytes by the peroxisome proliferator-activated receptor-γ agonist rosiglitazone. Diabetologia 2006; 49(6): 1303-10.
[http://dx.doi.org/10.1007/s00125-006-0228-1] [PMID: 16609881]

[157]   Bjursell M, Ahnmark A, Bohlooly-Y M, *et al.* Opposing effects of adiponectin receptors 1 and 2 on energy metabolism. Diabetes 2007; 56(3): 583-93.
[http://dx.doi.org/10.2337/db06-1432] [PMID: 17327425]

[158] Yamauchi T, Kamon J, Ito Y, *et al.* Cloning of adiponectin receptors that mediate antidiabetic metabolic effects. Nature 2003; 423(6941): 762-9.
[http://dx.doi.org/10.1038/nature01705] [PMID: 12802337]

[159] Mora-García GG, Ruiz-Díaz MS, Espitia-Almeida F, Gómez-Camargo D. Variations in ADIPOR1 but not ADIPOR2 are associated with hypertriglyceridemia and diabetes in an admixed Latin American population. Rev Diabet Stud 2017; 14(2-3): 311-28.
[http://dx.doi.org/10.1900/RDS.2017.14.311] [PMID: 29145541]

[160] Civitarese AE, Jenkinson CP, Richardson D, *et al.* Adiponectin receptors gene expression and insulin sensitivity in non-diabetic Mexican Americans with or without a family history of Type 2 diabetes. Diabetologia 2004; 47(5): 816-20.
[http://dx.doi.org/10.1007/s00125-004-1359-x] [PMID: 15105989]

[161] Tanabe H, Fujii Y, Okada-Iwabu M, *et al.* Crystal structures of the human adiponectin receptors. Nature 2015; 520(7547): 312-6.
[http://dx.doi.org/10.1038/nature14301] [PMID: 25855295]

[162] Yamauchi T, Kadowaki T. Adiponectin receptor as a key player in healthy longevity and obesity-related diseases. Cell Metab 2013; 17(2): 185-96.
[http://dx.doi.org/10.1016/j.cmet.2013.01.001] [PMID: 23352188]

[163] Achari A, Jain S. Adiponectin, a therapeutic target for obesity, diabetes, and endothelial dysfunction. Int J Mol Sci 2017; 18(6): 1321.
[http://dx.doi.org/10.3390/ijms18061321] [PMID: 28635626]

[164] Yamauchi T, Nio Y, Maki T, *et al.* Targeted disruption of AdipoR1 and AdipoR2 causes abrogation of adiponectin binding and metabolic actions. Nat Med 2007; 13(3): 332-9.
[http://dx.doi.org/10.1038/nm1557] [PMID: 17268472]

[165] Asahara N, Okada-Iwabu M, Iwabu M, *et al.* A monoclonal antibody activating AdipoR for type 2 diabetes and nonalcoholic steatohepatitis. Sci Adv 2023; 9(45): eadg4216.
[http://dx.doi.org/10.1126/sciadv.adg4216] [PMID: 37948516]

[166] Ma OKF, Ronsisvalle S, Basile L, *et al.* Identification of a novel adiponectin receptor and opioid receptor dual acting agonist as a potential treatment for diabetic neuropathy. Biomed Pharmacother 2023; 158: 114141.
[http://dx.doi.org/10.1016/j.biopha.2022.114141] [PMID: 36542987]

[167] Okada-Iwabu M, Yamauchi T, Iwabu M, *et al.* A small-molecule AdipoR agonist for type 2 diabetes and short life in obesity. Nature 2013; 503(7477): 493-9.
[http://dx.doi.org/10.1038/nature12656] [PMID: 24172895]

[168] Guan HP, Xiong Y. Learn from failures and stay hopeful to GPR40, a GPCR target with robust efficacy, for therapy of metabolic disorders. Front Pharmacol 2022; 13: 1043828.
[http://dx.doi.org/10.3389/fphar.2022.1043828] [PMID: 36386134]

[169] Burant CF. Activation of GPR40 as a therapeutic target for the treatment of type 2 diabetes. Diabetes Care 2013; 36(Suppl 2) (Suppl. 2): S175-9.
[http://dx.doi.org/10.2337/dcS13-2037] [PMID: 23882043]

[170] Ferdaoussi M, Bergeron V, Zarrouki B, *et al.* G protein-coupled receptor (GPR)40-dependent potentiation of insulin secretion in mouse islets is mediated by protein kinase D1. Diabetologia 2012; 55(10): 2682-92.
[http://dx.doi.org/10.1007/s00125-012-2650-x] [PMID: 22820510]

[171] Chen C, Li H, Long YQ. GPR40 agonists for the treatment of type 2 diabetes mellitus: The biological characteristics and the chemical space. Bioorg Med Chem Lett 2016; 26(23): 5603-12.
[http://dx.doi.org/10.1016/j.bmcl.2016.10.074] [PMID: 27825762]

[172] Cione E, Caroleo MC, Kagechika H, Manetti F. Pharmacophore-guided repurposing of fibrates and retinoids as GPR40 allosteric ligands with activity on insulin release. J Enzyme Inhib Med Chem

2021; 36(1): 377-83.
[http://dx.doi.org/10.1080/14756366.2020.1864629] [PMID: 33525941]

[173] Liu JJ, Wang Y, Ma Z, *et al.* Optimization of GPR40 agonists for type 2 diabetes. ACS Med Chem Lett 2014; 5(5): 517-21.
[http://dx.doi.org/10.1021/ml400501x] [PMID: 24900872]

[174] DiStefano JK, Watanabe RM. Pharmacogenetics of Anti-diabetes drugs. Pharmaceuticals (Basel) 2010; 3(8): 2610-46.
[http://dx.doi.org/10.3390/ph3082610] [PMID: 20936101]

[175] Chen S, Zhou J, Xi M, Jia Y, Wong Y, Zhao J, *et al.* Pharmacogenetic variation and metformin response. Curr Drug Metab. 2013 Dec;14(10):1070–82. doi: 10.2174/13892002146661131211153933. PMID: 24329113.

[176] Grzybowska M, Bober J, Olszewska M. Metformin - mechanisms of action and use for the treatment of type 2 diabetes mellitus. Postepy Hig Med Dosw 2011; 65: 277-85.
[http://dx.doi.org/10.5604/17322693.941655] [PMID: 21677353]

[177] Hu C. Pharmacogenomics in type 2 diabetes management: towards personalized medicine. J Transl Med 2012; 10(S2): A19.
[http://dx.doi.org/10.1186/1479-5876-10-S2-A19]

[178] Mannino GC, Andreozzi F, Sesti G. Pharmacogenetics of type 2 diabetes mellitus, the route toward tailored medicine. Diabetes Metab Res Rev 2019; 35(3): e3109.
[http://dx.doi.org/10.1002/dmrr.3109] [PMID: 30515958]

[179] Sarah EH, El Omri N, Ibrahimi A, El Jaoudi R. Metabolic and genetic studies of glimepiride and metformin and their association with type 2 diabetes. Gene Rep 2020; 21: 100787.
[http://dx.doi.org/10.1016/j.genrep.2020.100787]

[180] Singh S, Usman K, Banerjee M. Pharmacogenetic studies update in type 2 diabetes mellitus. World J Diabetes 2016; 7(15): 302-15.
[http://dx.doi.org/10.4239/wjd.v7.i15.302] [PMID: 27555891]

[181] Pearson ER. Personalized medicine in diabetes: The role of 'omics' and biomarkers. Diabet Med 2016; 33(6): 712-7.
[http://dx.doi.org/10.1111/dme.13075] [PMID: 26802434]

[182] Imamovic Kadric S, Kulo Cesic A, Dujić T. Pharmacogenetics of new classes of antidiabetic drugs. Bosn J Basic Med Sci 2021; 21(6): 659-71.
[http://dx.doi.org/10.17305/bjbms.2021.5646] [PMID: 33974529]

[183] Topić E. The role of pharmacogenetics in the treatment of diabetes mellitus. J Med Biochem 2014; 33(1): 58-70.
[http://dx.doi.org/10.2478/jomb-2013-0045]

[184] Cresci S. Pharmacogenetics of the PPAR genes and cardiovascular disease. Pharmacogenomics 2007; 8(11): 1581-95.
[http://dx.doi.org/10.2217/14622416.8.11.1581] [PMID: 18034623]

[185] Hossain U, Das AK, Ghosh S, Sil PC. An overview on the role of bioactive α-glucosidase inhibitors in ameliorating diabetic complications. Food Chem Toxicol 2020; 145: 111738.
[http://dx.doi.org/10.1016/j.fct.2020.111738] [PMID: 32916220]

[186] Coleman RL, Scott CAB, Lang Z, Bethel MA, Tuomilehto J, Holman RR. Meta-analysis of the impact of alpha-glucosidase inhibitors on incident diabetes and cardiovascular outcomes. Cardiovasc Diabetol 2019; 18(1): 135.
[http://dx.doi.org/10.1186/s12933-019-0933-y] [PMID: 31623625]

[187] Van de Laar FA, Lucassen PLBJ, Akkermans RP, *et al.* Alpha-glucosidase inhibitors for type 2 diabetes mellitus. Cochrane Database Syst Rev 2009.
[http://dx.doi.org/10.1002/14651858.CD003639.pub2]

[188]   Riyaphan J, Pham DC, Leong MK, Weng CF. *In silico* approaches to identify polyphenol compounds as α-glucosidase and α-amylase inhibitors against type-2 diabetes. Biomolecules 2021; 11(12): 1877.
[http://dx.doi.org/10.3390/biom11121877] [PMID: 34944521]

[189]   Kashtoh H, Baek KH. Recent updates on phytoconstituent alpha-glucosidase inhibitors: An approach towards the treatment of type two diabetes. Plants 2022; 11(20): 2722.
[http://dx.doi.org/10.3390/plants11202722] [PMID: 36297746]

[190]   McKinley BJ, Santiago M, Pak C, Nguyen N, Zhong Q. Pneumatosis intestinalis induced by alpha-glucosidase inhibitors in patients with diabetes mellitus. J Clin Med 2022; 11(19): 5918.
[http://dx.doi.org/10.3390/jcm11195918] [PMID: 36233785]

[191]   Pathak R, Bridgeman MB, Bridgeman MB. Dipeptidyl peptidase-4 (DPP-4) inhibitors in the management of diabetes. P and T; 35

[192]   Liu D, Jin B, Chen W, Yun P. Dipeptidyl peptidase 4 (DPP-4) inhibitors and cardiovascular outcomes in patients with Type 2 Diabetes Mellitus (T2DM): A systematic review and meta-analysis. BMC Pharmacol Toxicol 2019; 20(1): 15.
[http://dx.doi.org/10.1186/s40360-019-0293-y] [PMID: 30832701]

[193]   Sharma P, Anikhindi A, Kumar A, *et al.* Dipeptidyl peptidase 4 (DPP-4) inhibitors in patients with cirrhosis and diabetes. J Clin Exp Hepatol 2023; 13: S152.
[http://dx.doi.org/10.1016/j.jceh.2023.07.128]

[194]   Kristin E. Dipeptidyl peptidase 4 (DPP-4) inhibitors for the treatment of type 2 diabetes mellitus. *J thee Med Sci.* Berkala Ilmu Kedokteran 2016; 48
[http://dx.doi.org/10.19106/JMedSci004802201606]

[195]   Wang X, Zheng P, Huang G, Yang L, Zhou Z. Dipeptidyl peptidase-4(DPP-4) inhibitors: Promising new agents for autoimmune diabetes. Clin Exp Med 2018; 18(4): 473-80.
[http://dx.doi.org/10.1007/s10238-018-0519-0] [PMID: 30022375]

[196]   Hamrick I, Goblirsch MJ, Tuan WJ, Beckham F. Transitioning from insulin to dipeptidyl-peptidase 4 (DPP-4) inhibitors for type 2 diabetes. Geriatr Nurs 2022; 46: 86-9.
[http://dx.doi.org/10.1016/j.gerinurse.2022.04.023] [PMID: 35613488]

[197]   Richter B, Bandeira-Echtler E, Bergerhoff K, Lerch C. Dipeptidyl peptidase-4 (DPP-4) inhibitors for type 2 diabetes mellitus. Cochrane Libr 2008; 2010(1): CD006739.
[http://dx.doi.org/10.1002/14651858.CD006739.pub2] [PMID: 18425967]

[198]   Rathmann W, Bongaerts B. Pharmacogenetics of novel glucose-lowering drugs. Diabetologia 2021; 64(6): 1201-12.
[http://dx.doi.org/10.1007/s00125-021-05402-w] [PMID: 33594477]

[199]   Samoilova IG, Stankova AE, Matveeva MV, *et al.* Pharmacogenetics of glucagon-like peptide-1 agonists in the treatment of type 2 diabetes mellitus. Russian Journal of Preventive Medicine 2023; 26(12): 95.
[http://dx.doi.org/10.17116/profmed20232612195]

[200]   Jakhar K, Vaishnavi S, Kaur P, Singh P, Munshi A. Pharmacogenomics of GLP-1 receptor agonists: Focus on pharmacological profile. Eur J Pharmacol 2022; 936: 175356.
[http://dx.doi.org/10.1016/j.ejphar.2022.175356] [PMID: 36330902]

[201]   Svendsen B, Capozzi ME, Nui J, *et al.* Pharmacological antagonism of the incretin system protects against diet-induced obesity. Mol Metab 2020; 32: 44-55.
[http://dx.doi.org/10.1016/j.molmet.2019.11.018] [PMID: 32029229]

[202]   Wang JY, Wang QW, Yang XY, *et al.* GLP−1 receptor agonists for the treatment of obesity: Role as a promising approach. Front Endocrinol (Lausanne) 2023; 14: 1085799.
[http://dx.doi.org/10.3389/fendo.2023.1085799] [PMID: 36843578]

[203]   Klen J, Dolžan V. Glucagon-like peptide-1 receptor agonists in the management of type 2 diabetes

mellitus and obesity: The impact of pharmacological properties and genetic factors. Int J Mol Sci 2022; 23(7): 3451.
[http://dx.doi.org/10.3390/ijms23073451] [PMID: 35408810]

[204] Tarasova L, Kalnina I, Geldnere K, *et al.* Association of genetic variation in the organic cation transporters OCT1, OCT2 and multidrug and toxin extrusion 1 transporter protein genes with the gastrointestinal side effects and lower BMI in metformin-treated type 2 diabetes patients. Pharmacogenet Genomics 2012; 22(9): 659-66.
[http://dx.doi.org/10.1097/FPC.0b013e3283561666] [PMID: 22735389]

[205] Manolopoulos VG, Ragia G, Tavridou A. Pharmacogenomics of oral antidiabetic medications: Current data and pharmacoepigenomic perspective. Pharmacogenomics 2011; 12(8): 1161-91.
[http://dx.doi.org/10.2217/pgs.11.65] [PMID: 21843065]

[206] Aquilante CL, Lam YWF. The role of pharmacogenomics in diabetes, HIV infection, and pain management. In: Pharmacogenomics: Challenges and Opportunities in Therapeutic Implementation. 2013.
[http://dx.doi.org/10.1016/B978-0-12-391918-2.00007-X]

[207] Markowicz-Piasecka M, Huttunen KM, Mateusiak L, Mikiciuk-Olasik E, Sikora J. Is metformin a perfect drug? Updates in pharmacokinetics and pharmacodynamics. Curr Pharm Des 2017; 23(17): 2532-50.
[http://dx.doi.org/10.2174/1381612822666161201152941] [PMID: 27908266]

[208] Mohseni S, Tabatabaei Malazy O, Bandarian F, Larijani B. Pharmacogenomics of glibenclamide in patients with type 2 diabetes mellitus: a systematic review. Koomesh. 2022;24(2):e152659.

[209] Kalra S, Das AK, Bajaj S, *et al.* Utility of precision medicine in the management of diabetes: Expert opinion from an international panel. Diabetes Ther 2020; 11(2): 411-22.
[http://dx.doi.org/10.1007/s13300-019-00753-5] [PMID: 31916214]

[210] Dhawan D, Padh H. Genetic variations in TCF7L2 influence therapeutic response to sulfonylureas in Indian diabetics. Diabetes Res Clin Pract 2016; 121: 35-40.
[http://dx.doi.org/10.1016/j.diabres.2016.08.018] [PMID: 27639123]

[211] Maruthur NM, Gribble MO, Bennett WL, *et al.* The pharmacogenetics of type 2 diabetes: A systematic review. Diabetes Care 2014; 37(3): 876-86.
[http://dx.doi.org/10.2337/dc13-1276] [PMID: 24558078]

[212] Kuate Defo A, Bakula V, Pisaturo A, Labos C, Wing SS, Daskalopoulou SS. Diabetes, antidiabetic medications and risk of dementia: A systematic umbrella review and meta-analysis. Diabetes Obes Metab 2024; 26(2): 441-62.
[http://dx.doi.org/10.1111/dom.15331] [PMID: 37869901]

[213] Rudovich N, Möhlig M, Otto B, *et al.* Effect of meglitinides on postprandial ghrelin secretion pattern in type 2 diabetes mellitus. Diabetes Technol Ther 2010; 12(1): 57-64.
[http://dx.doi.org/10.1089/dia.2009.0129] [PMID: 20082586]

[214] Nasykhova YA, Tonyan ZN, Mikhailova AA, Danilova MM, Glotov AS. Pharmacogenetics of type 2 diabetes—progress and prospects. Int J Mol Sci 2020; 21(18): 6842.
[http://dx.doi.org/10.3390/ijms21186842] [PMID: 32961860]

[215] Pacanowski MA, Hopley CW, Aquilante CL. Interindividual variability in oral antidiabetic drug disposition and response: The role of drug transporter polymorphisms. Expert Opin Drug Metab Toxicol 2008; 4(5): 529-44.
[http://dx.doi.org/10.1517/17425255.4.5.529] [PMID: 18484913]

[216] Grant JS, Graven LJ. Progressing from metformin to sulfonylureas or meglitinides. Workplace Health Saf 2016; 64(9): 433-9.
[http://dx.doi.org/10.1177/2165079916644263] [PMID: 27621259]

[217] Blanquez Martinez D, Hayon Ponce M, Casas Hidalgo I, *et al.* Pharmacogenetics of oral antidiabetic

treatment in type 2 diabetes. Int J Clin Pharm 2019; 41: 289-383. 47th ESCP Symposium on Clinical Pharmacy: Personalised pharmacy care, 24–26 October 2018, Belfast, Northern Ireland.
[http://dx.doi.org/10.1007/s11096-018-0759-9]

[218]   Rizos CV, Kei A, Elisaf MS. The current role of thiazolidinediones in diabetes management. Arch Toxicol 2016; 90(8): 1861-81.
[http://dx.doi.org/10.1007/s00204-016-1737-4] [PMID: 27165418]

[219]   Ji X, Zhang W, Yin L, *et al.* The potential roles of post-translational modifications of PPARγ in treating diabetes. Biomolecules 2022; 12(12): 1832.
[http://dx.doi.org/10.3390/biom12121832] [PMID: 36551260]

[220]   Soccio RE, Chen ER, Lazar MA. Thiazolidinediones and the promise of insulin sensitization in type 2 diabetes. Cell Metab 2014; 20(4): 573-91.
[http://dx.doi.org/10.1016/j.cmet.2014.08.005] [PMID: 25242225]

[221]   Lebovitz HE. Thiazolidinediones: The forgotten diabetes medications. Curr Diab Rep 2019; 19(12): 151.
[http://dx.doi.org/10.1007/s11892-019-1270-y] [PMID: 31776781]

[222]   Xue CY, Zhou MQ, Zheng QY, *et al.* Thiazolidinediones play a positive role in the vascular endothelium and inhibit plaque progression in diabetic patients with coronary atherosclerosis: A systematic review and meta-analysis. Front Cardiovasc Med 2022; 9: 1043406.
[http://dx.doi.org/10.3389/fcvm.2022.1043406] [PMID: 36523368]

[223]   Nanjan MJ, Mohammed M, Prashantha Kumar BR, Chandrasekar MJN. Thiazolidinediones as antidiabetic agents: A critical review. Bioorg Chem 2018; 77: 548-67.
[http://dx.doi.org/10.1016/j.bioorg.2018.02.009] [PMID: 29475164]

[224]   Kumari D. Exploring the potential benefits and risks of 2,4-thiazolidinediones (TZDs) in the management of diabetes and related conditions. J Pharmacol Drug Deliv 2023.
[http://dx.doi.org/10.59462/JPDD.1.1.101]

[225]   Rizzo MR, Di Meo I, Polito R, *et al.* Cognitive impairment and type 2 diabetes mellitus: Focus of SGLT2 inhibitors treatment. Pharmacol Res 2022; 176: 106062.
[http://dx.doi.org/10.1016/j.phrs.2022.106062] [PMID: 35017046]

[226]   Thomas MC, Neuen BL, Twigg SM, Cooper ME, Badve SV. SGLT2 inhibitors for patients with type 2 diabetes and CKD: A narrative review. Endocr Connect 2023; 12(8): e230005.
[http://dx.doi.org/10.1530/EC-23-0005] [PMID: 37159343]

[227]   Bays H. Sodium glucose co-transporter type 2 (SGLT2) inhibitors: Targeting the kidney to improve glycemic control in diabetes mellitus. Diabetes Ther 2013; 4(2): 195-220.
[http://dx.doi.org/10.1007/s13300-013-0042-y] [PMID: 24142577]

[228]   Bailey CJ, Day C, Bellary S. Renal protection with SGLT2 inhibitors: Effects in acute and chronic kidney disease. Curr Diab Rep 2022; 22(1): 39-52.
[http://dx.doi.org/10.1007/s11892-021-01442-z] [PMID: 35113333]

[229]   Wilding JPH. The role of the kidneys in glucose homeostasis in type 2 diabetes: Clinical implications and therapeutic significance through sodium glucose co-transporter 2 inhibitors. Metabolism 2014; 63(10): 1228-37.
[http://dx.doi.org/10.1016/j.metabol.2014.06.018] [PMID: 25104103]

[230]   Kaur P, Behera BS, Singh S, Munshi A. "The pharmacological profile of SGLT2 inhibitors: Focus on mechanistic aspects and pharmacogenomics". Eur J Pharmacol 2021; 904: 174169.
[http://dx.doi.org/10.1016/j.ejphar.2021.174169] [PMID: 33984301]

[231]   Kaur P, Kotru S, Tuteja L, Ludhiadch A, Munshi A. Role of SGLT2 inhibitors in diabetes management: Focus on HbA1c levels, weight loss and genetic variation. Journal of Medical and Health Studies 2023; 4(4): 187-96.
[http://dx.doi.org/10.32996/jmhs.2023.4.4.20]

[232] Marks J. Insulin analogues. Postgrad Med 2002; 112(5) (Suppl Designer): 8-12.
[http://dx.doi.org/10.3810/pgm.1997.02.157] [PMID: 19667599]

[233] Sebastian SA, Co EL, Mehendale M, Hameed M. Insulin analogs in the treatment of type II diabetes and future perspectives. Dis Mon 2023; 69(3): 101417.
[http://dx.doi.org/10.1016/j.disamonth.2022.101417] [PMID: 35487767]

[234] Chen W, Lu J, Plum-Mörschel L, *et al.* Pharmacokinetic and pharmacodynamic bioequivalence of Gan & Lee insulin analogues aspart (rapilin®), lispro (prandilin®) and glargine (basalin®) with EU - und US-SOURCED reference insulins. Diabetes Obes Metab 2023; 25(12): 3817-25.
[http://dx.doi.org/10.1111/dom.15281] [PMID: 37735841]

[235] Insulin-aspart/insulin-glargine/insulin-lispro React Wkly 1804.
[http://dx.doi.org/10.1007/s40278-020-78588-9]

[236] Hemkens LG, Grouven U, Bender R, *et al.* Risk of malignancies in patients with diabetes treated with human insulin or insulin analogues: A cohort study. Diabetologia 2009; 52(9): 1732-44.
[http://dx.doi.org/10.1007/s00125-009-1418-4] [PMID: 19565214]

[237] Garige M, Ghosh S, Roelofs B, Rao VA, Sourbier C. Protocol to assess the biological activity of insulin glargine, insulin lispro, and insulin aspart *in vitro*. Methods Protoc 2023; 6(2): 33.
[http://dx.doi.org/10.3390/mps6020033] [PMID: 37104015]

[238] Støy J, De Franco E, Ye H, Park SY, Bell GI, Hattersley AT. In celebration of a century with insulin – Update of insulin gene mutations in diabetes. Mol Metab 2021; 52: 101280.
[http://dx.doi.org/10.1016/j.molmet.2021.101280] [PMID: 34174481]

[239] Panda C, Kumar S, Gupta S, Pandey LM. Structural, kinetic, and thermodynamic aspects of insulin aggregation. Phys Chem Chem Phys 2023; 25(36): 24195-213.
[http://dx.doi.org/10.1039/D3CP03103A] [PMID: 37674360]

[240] Sherwin RS, Kramer KJ, Tobin JD, *et al.* A model of the kinetics of insulin in man. J Clin Invest 1974; 53(5): 1481-92.
[http://dx.doi.org/10.1172/JCI107697] [PMID: 4856884]

[241] Morettini M, Palumbo MC, Göbl C, *et al.* Mathematical model of insulin kinetics accounting for the amino acids effect during a mixed meal tolerance test. Front Endocrinol (Lausanne) 2022; 13: 966305.
[http://dx.doi.org/10.3389/fendo.2022.966305] [PMID: 36187117]

[242] Doskicz J. The 6 types of insulin: a guide to regular, short-, and long-acting insulins. Healthline 2022. Available at: www.healthline.com/health/diabetes/types-of-insulin

[243] Racsa PN, Meah Y, Ellis JJ, Saverno KR. Comparative effectiveness of rapid-acting insulins in adults with diabetes. J Manag Care Spec Pharm 2017; 23(3): 291-8.
[http://dx.doi.org/10.18553/jmcp.2017.23.3.291] [PMID: 28230457]

[244] De Block CEM, Van Cauwenberghe J, Bochanen N, Dirinck E. RAPID-ACTING insulin analogues: Theory and best clinical practice in type 1 and type 2 diabetes. Diabetes Obes Metab 2022; 24(S1) (Suppl. 1): 63-74.
[http://dx.doi.org/10.1111/dom.14713] [PMID: 35403348]

[245] Siebenhofer A, Plank J, Berghold A, *et al.* Short acting insulin analogues versus regular human insulin in patients with diabetes mellitus. Cochrane Libr 2006; (2): CD003287.
[http://dx.doi.org/10.1002/14651858.CD003287.pub4] [PMID: 16625575]

[246] Fullerton B, Siebenhofer A, Jeitler K, *et al.* Short-acting insulin analogues versus regular human insulin for adults with type 1 diabetes mellitus. Cochrane Database of Systematic Reviews 2016.
[http://dx.doi.org/10.1002/14651858.CD012161]

[247] Fullerton B, Siebenhofer A, Jeitler K, *et al.* Short-acting insulin analogues versus regular human insulin for adult, non-pregnant persons with type 2 diabetes mellitus. Cochrane Database of Systematic Reviews 2018.

[http://dx.doi.org/10.1002/14651858.CD013228]

[248] Vardi M, Jacobson E, Nini A, Bitterman H. Intermediate acting versus long acting insulin for type 1 diabetes mellitus. Cochrane Libr 2008; 2008(3): CD006297.
[http://dx.doi.org/10.1002/14651858.CD006297.pub2] [PMID: 18646147]

[249] Dedov II, Shestakova M V. Insulin degludec is a new ultra-long-acting insulin analogue Diabetes Mellit 2014.
[http://dx.doi.org/10.14341/DM2014291-104]

[250] Davis CS, Fleming JW, Malinowski SS, Brown MA, Fleming LW. Ultra-long-acting insulins: A review of efficacy, safety, and implications for practice. J Am Assoc Nurse Pract 2018; 30(7): 373-80.
[http://dx.doi.org/10.1097/JXX.0000000000000076] [PMID: 29979295]

[251] Swain J, Jena S, Manglunia A, Singh J. The journey of insulin over 100 years. Journal of Diabetology 2022; 13(1): 8-15.
[http://dx.doi.org/10.4103/jod.jod_100_21]

[252] Søeborg T, Rasmussen CH, Mosekilde E, Colding-Jørgensen M. Absorption kinetics of insulin after subcutaneous administration. Eur J Pharm Sci 2009; 36(1): 78-90.
[http://dx.doi.org/10.1016/j.ejps.2008.10.018] [PMID: 19028573]

[253] Ismail L, Materwala H, Al Kaabi J. Association of risk factors with type 2 diabetes: A systematic review. Comput Struct Biotechnol J 2021; 19: 1759-85.
[http://dx.doi.org/10.1016/j.csbj.2021.03.003] [PMID: 33897980]

[254] Teh WT, Teede HJ, Paul E, Harrison CL, Wallace EM, Allan C. Risk factors for gestational diabetes mellitus: Implications for the application of screening guidelines. Aust N Z J Obstet Gynaecol 2011; 51(1): 26-30.
[http://dx.doi.org/10.1111/j.1479-828X.2011.01292.x] [PMID: 21299505]

[255] Weihrauch-Blüher S, Wiegand S. Risk factors and implications of childhood obesity. Curr Obes Rep 2018; 7(4): 254-9.
[http://dx.doi.org/10.1007/s13679-018-0320-0] [PMID: 30315490]

[256] Garcia-Compean D, Jaquez-Quintana JO, Gonzalez-Gonzalez JA, Maldonado-Garza H. Liver cirrhosis and diabetes: Risk factors, pathophysiology, clinical implications and management. World J Gastroenterol 2009; 15(3): 280-8.
[http://dx.doi.org/10.3748/wjg.15.280] [PMID: 19140227]

[257] Wicklow B, Retnakaran R. Gestational diabetes mellitus and its implications across the life span. Diabetes Metab J 2023; 47(3): 333-44.
[http://dx.doi.org/10.4093/dmj.2022.0348] [PMID: 36750271]

[258] Wu Y, Ding Y, Tanaka Y, Zhang W. Risk factors contributing to type 2 diabetes and recent advances in the treatment and prevention. Int J Med Sci 2014; 11(11): 1185-200.
[http://dx.doi.org/10.7150/ijms.10001] [PMID: 25249787]

CHAPTER 3

Existing Technologies in Diabetes Care

Abstract: Millions of people worldwide suffer from diabetes, a chronic metabolic disease that needs to be accurately and consistently managed. The disorder is being treated by technological developments that improve blood glucose management. An overview of the main technologies used to manage diabetes is given in this chapter, including insulin pumps, artificial pancreas systems, and Continuous Glucose Monitoring (CGM) devices. Multiple insulin injections are no longer necessary thanks to real-time blood glucose regulation. There is a detailed discussion of emerging tools, such as *in silico* sensors, which anticipate glucose dynamics using computational models. They guarantee the best possible insulin delivery based on information gathered from the effective application of closed-loop control algorithms. Additionally, the use of AI and machine learning will further improve the efficacy of individualized therapy, and simple, accurate, and portable insulin pens are discussed as diabetes care solutions. Even with the advances in technology, issues like cost, availability, and data security continue to be significant. Nevertheless, a bright future is anticipated, with advances significantly improving patient outcomes.

Keywords: Artificial pancreas, CGM, Diabetes, *In silico*, Insulin pump, Insulin pens.

INTRODUCTION

Diabetes mellitus is a long-term metabolic disease that is on the rise and requires accurate and constant management to avoid complications and improve life quality. The burden diabetes imposes necessitates the development of new technologies for blood glucose regulation and patient care. The approach to diabetes treatment is changing with the introduction of new technology, moving from manual, labor-intensive methods to more advanced automation. This chapter gives an account of the current approaches in diabetes care and management, including insulin pumps, artificial pancreas systems, Continuous Glucose Monitoring (CGM) devices, and *in silico* sensors.

In this chapter, we explore how novel blood glucose regulation technologies have eliminated the requirement for insulin injections, considerably simplifying the management of the disorder. *In silico* sensors now equipped with computational

Darshna M. Joshi, Hardik Bhatt & Himanshu K. Patel

models can forecast blood glucose shifts in real-time, leading to optimized insulin delivery and timely intervention. Moreover, with the development of Artificial Intelligence (AI) and Machine Learning (ML) algorithms, treatment plans can be optimized and even further personalized, which can lead to better patient outcomes with more intelligent and responsive care.

Additionally, the discussion also tackles the increasing uptake of insulin pens as they make diabetes management more convenient and effective. While the advancements in technology tailored for diabetes are encouraging, issues such as affordability, availability, and cybersecurity persist as significant challenges. Nonetheless, the advancements in caring for diabetes patients seem promising as continued development will likely help mitigate these issues and improve the experiences of patients around the world. This section serves to prepare the reader for the ways in which such neo-technologies are changing diabetes care for the better, providing those suffering from this disease with greater optimism around an otherwise dire condition.

GLUCOSE MONITORS, INSULIN PUMPS, AND ARTIFICIAL PANCREAS SYSTEMS: AN OVERVIEW

The global prevalence of diabetes has increased continuously in the past decades. As a result, it has become more important to focus on the advancements that take place in diabetes technologies. In addition to that, it is necessary that the technologies reach all the people in need on time and in a cost-effective manner [1 - 3]. Despite the advancements in technology, the life span of diabetic patients is drastically reducing these days. Glucose monitors, insulin pumps, and artificial pancreas are the most commonly used tools for the management of diabetes. These tools help in enhancing the quality of life of diabetic patients. It also provides accurate and precise glucose control. This section will give an overview of these three most useful tools for diabetes management [4 - 9].

Continuous Glucose Monitoring (CGM) systems are used for obtaining a timely measure of glucose and, hence, help in providing data for taking relevant action based on sugar levels in the body to manage insulin, plan diets, and physical activity. Throughout the day and night, one can easily observe the blood sugar levels with the help of CGM systems.

A CGM mainly consists of three parts, as shown in Fig.(**1**):

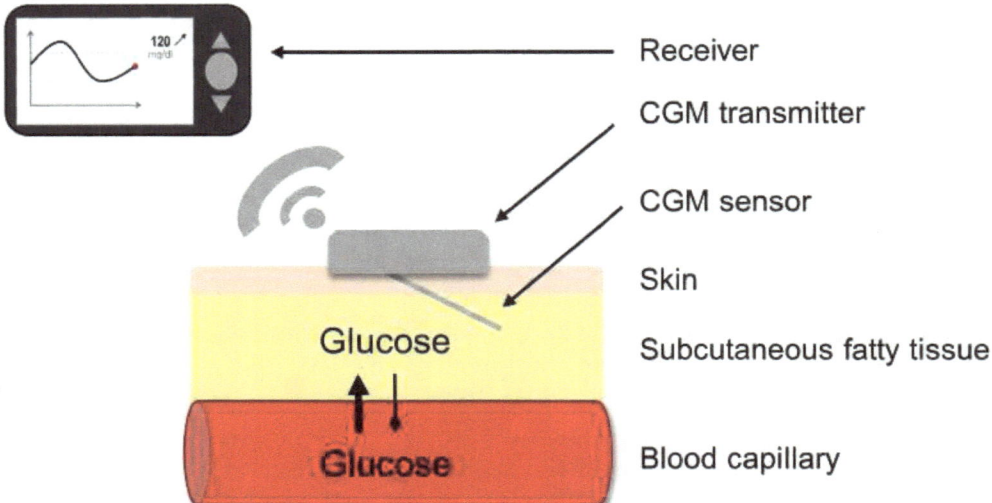

Fig. (1). Continuous glucose monitoring system.

1. **Sensor:** A small piece of material is placed on/under the skin, usually on the belly or arm. It is a disposable sensor. It helps with the estimation of glucose level in the interstitial fluid (fluid in the spaces around your cells). The sensor keeps track of the sugar level throughout the day at regular intervals. It is necessary to replace the sensor at specific times, like weekly or more often, based on the quality and capacity of the sensor used.
2. **Transmitter:** The data that is sensed by the sensor is then transmitted wirelessly to a device where one can view it. The transmitters are reusable and can be attached to various sensors.
3. **Software program:** Configured smart devices like phones, insulin pumps, or receivers receive the information transmitted by the transmitter and take necessary action to guide the diabetic patient for the management of diabetes.

CGMs are used to plan diets, workouts, and other medications in a smooth manner. The advancements in CGM also provide a graphical representation and alerts regarding the status of glucose levels, whether they are rising or falling. There is a drastic reduction in finger-prick tests observed with the introduction of CGM. However, it is important that when CGM gives an alert, one needs to verify it using a finger prick test for precise confirmation. The difficulty observed while using CGM is the replacement cycle of the sensors at specific times, skin irritation caused by sensor placement adhesives, and the cost associated with the same. Also, some medications used for diabetes may interfere with the accuracy of CGM. However, the difficulties are mitigated by real-time glucose monitoring, alert systems, and the ability to share data with healthcare providers for faster treatment. Dexcom G6, Freestyle Libre, and Medtronic Guardian Connect are some CGM systems that are most popular for diabetes management [4 - 6, 10 - 12].

Another important thing about CGM is the clinical trials carried out for the evaluation of the safety and performance of new devices. It helps in the assessment of how the CGMs respond to reduce the complications associated with diabetes management in real-world settings in order to enhance the quality of life of individuals with diabetes [13 - 15].

An insulin pump is a small mechatronic wearable device that helps to deliver insulin at a selected rate, which helps in maintaining glucose levels for diabetics. The size of the pump is so comfortable that users can handle it with ease. With technological advancements, insulin pumps come with extra features like touchscreens, alarm alerts, and waterproofing. Also, some insulin pumps can communicate with CGMs and hence make decisions to maintain the delivery of insulin according to blood glucose levels in the body. An insulin pump serves as an alternative to the daily use of multiple insulin therapy injections. An insulin pump basically mimics the function of the pancreas in the body, which releases insulin when needed [16, 17].

Basically, there are two types of insulin pumps: Tubed and Tubeless. A tube (tethered) insulin pump consists of thin, long tubes. It connects the insulin pump to a cannula under the skin and delivers insulin. A flexible plastic tube (cannula) is inserted beneath the skin by tubeless insulin pumps, also known as patch pumps. However, the cannula and the insulin reservoir form a single "pod" that adheres to the skin. No external tubing is present. A handheld controller can be used to wirelessly operate the pump [18 - 20].

The design of the pump is determined based on the clinical requirements, such as treatment parameters and biocompatibility, user requirements like shape, size, and colour, and technical requirements like accuracy, reliability, and power consumption. As the insulin pump becomes part of the body, a thoughtful design of the pump is particularly important. Insulin pumps are designed to deliver both basal and bolus doses as needed. A basal dose is a small amount of insulin delivered throughout the day, while a bolus dose is a high amount of insulin that is delivered during meals. Sometimes, a correction dose is also delivered when needed [20].

The basic block diagram of an insulin pump is shown in Fig.(**2**). The infusion set is the main link between the human body and the insulin pump. It consists of a soft material that does not react with the medication or the application site. It acts as the only source that can isolate the insulin pump from the body. The cartridge is the reservoir for insulin, from which insulin is delivered as needed with the help of a connected pump. It can be refilled as per the dosages recommended by the doctor. The processing module acts as the brain of the complete system. It helps command the delivery of insulin, as well as manage other communication tasks like generating alerts and notifications to the user. Furthermore, the complete system works seamlessly with the help of a power supply module that delivers power for 4-6 weeks without requiring recharging or battery replacement. The monitoring modules are used to monitor blood glucose levels in real time so that important decisions can be made accordingly [20].

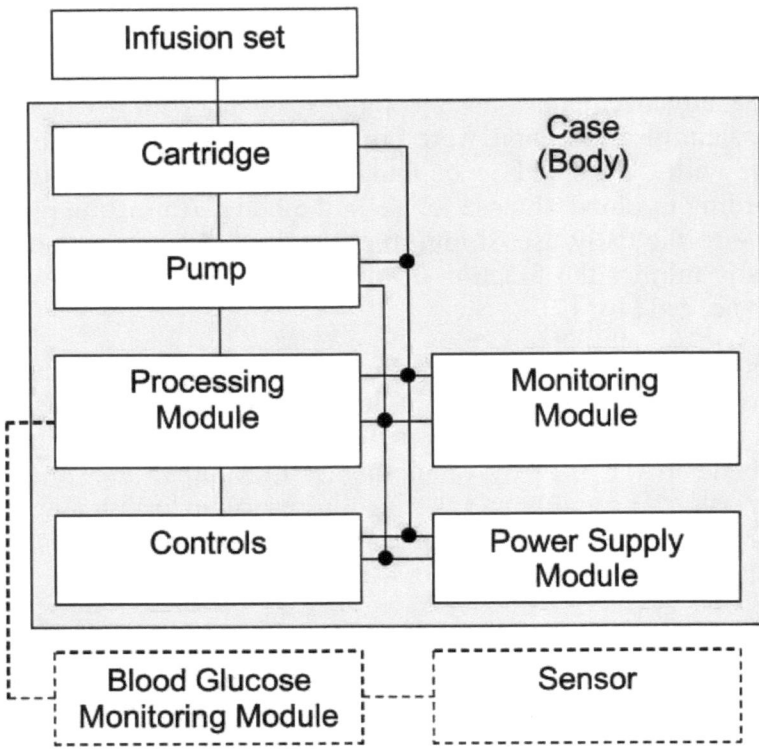

Fig. (2). Insulin pump unit.

The pancreas is an organ in the body that releases the hormone insulin in response to elevated blood sugar levels. When there is a disruption in this system, either insulin is not produced or it is insufficiently produced. This leads to the onset of diabetes. For the same reason, artificial pancreases are designed to regulate the delivery of insulin in people with pancreatic disorders. The artificial pancreas system mimics the regulation of blood glucose in the body like a healthy pancreas. It consists of CGM, a control algorithm, and an insulin infusion pump.

It regulates the insulin delivery in response to the blood glucose levels in the body. They are designed to provide robust glucose control with minimal patient intervention, as shown in Fig.(**3**) [21, 22].

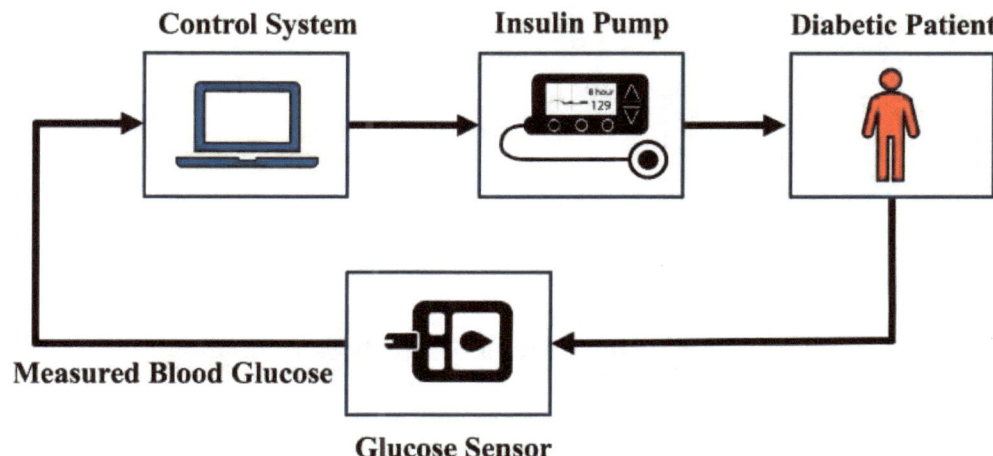

Fig. (3). Artificial pancreas device.

The successful artificial pancreas devices are those that have a robust control algorithm designed to respond to the elevated glucose levels in the body. The system gets affected by the lag time associated with the continuous glucose monitoring system. If the synchronization of the sensor, controller, and insulin pump is not maintained, there are chances of failure in blood glucose regulation in the body. Hence, the estimation of real-time parameters, clinical studies, and control techniques needs to be evaluated for designing and developing safe and efficient artificial pancreas device systems. The closed-loop control algorithm used for the artificial pancreas will be discussed in detail in the following sections [16, 21, 23 - 25].

Non-Invasive Glucose Monitoring: DiaMonTech's D-Pocket Device

Non-invasive glucose monitoring offers a groundbreaking solution for diabetes care, reducing the pain and inconvenience of traditional blood sampling methods. The D-Pocket by DiaMonTech is an innovative device designed to measure blood glucose levels without piercing the skin [26]. Compact and comparable in size to a modern smartphone, this portable tool employs mid-infrared quantum cascade laser spectroscopy to identify glucose molecules beneath the skin's surface [26]. Users simply place their finger on the device's sensor, which delivers glucose readings either on its display or *via* a connected smartphone application, making it ideal for convenient diabetes management on the move [26].

Clinical research on DiaMonTech's earlier model, the D-Base, conducted in 2020, showed that its accuracy rivals that of minimally invasive systems like Abbott's FreeStyle Libre in tests involving both diabetic and non-diabetic individuals [26]. The D-Pocket, tailored for personal use, is estimated to support around 50 measurements per battery charge [26]. DiaMonTech is also working on the D-Sensor, a future iteration aimed at continuous glucose monitoring every few minutes, with the added capability of tracking metrics like heart rate and blood pressure [26]. As of 2025, the D-Pocket remains in the development phase, awaiting CE approval and FDA clearance [26]. Despite its promise, non-invasive monitoring technologies face scrutiny due to past difficulties in achieving consistent accuracy, underscoring the importance of rigorous clinical validation to build confidence among users [26].

Insulin Delivery: Tandem t:slim X2 with Control-IQ Technology

The Tandem t:slim X2 insulin pump, equipped with Control-IQ technology, is a sophisticated hybrid closed-loop system that enhances blood sugar control in individuals with type 1 and type 2 diabetes [27, 28]. It pairs with Continuous Glucose Monitors (CGMs), such as the Dexcom G6 and G7, to dynamically adjust insulin delivery based on real-time glucose data and predictive algorithms [27, 28]. The Control-IQ system forecasts glucose levels 30 minutes before, modulating basal insulin to keep levels within a 112.5–160 mg/dL target range [27, 28]. It can escalate, reduce, or pause basal insulin and administer automatic correction boluses (up to one hourly) when glucose is projected to exceed 180 mg/dL, helping to prevent high blood sugar episodes [27, 28]. Additionally, it features a dedicated hypoglycemia prevention mechanism to reduce low glucose events, especially during sleep, aiming for morning glucose values between 100–120 mg/dL [27, 28].

Weighing 3.95 ounces (with battery and reservoir) and measuring 3.13 x 2 x 0.6 inches, the t:slim X2 is lightweight, equipped with a color touchscreen, and supports remote software updates for seamless feature enhancements [27, 28]. It is approved for use in type 1 diabetes patients aged 2 and older and type 2 diabetes patients aged 18 and older, using NovoLog or Humalog U-100 insulin [3]. Real-world studies have reported an increase in time in range (TIR, 70–180 mg/dL) from 70.5% to 73.0% among prior pump users, alongside notable reductions in HbA1c levels [29]. The system includes customizable settings for activities like sleep or exercise, offering tailored glucose management [27, 28]. However, users must manually administer meal boluses and maintain skills like carbohydrate counting [27, 28]. Smartphone integration enables discreet bolus delivery *via* mobile apps [27, 28]. The device is not suitable for pregnant females, those on dialysis, or patients using hydroxyurea, and requires a minimum daily insulin dose of 5 units [27, 28].

In Silico Modeling for Exogenous and Endogenous Insulin Differentiation

Cutting-edge in silico modeling techniques have been developed to separate exogenous (externally administered) and endogenous (body-produced) insulin in the bloodstream, providing valuable insights into optimizing diabetes treatments, including novel methods like inhaled insulin [29]. These models use dynamic simulations to analyze insulin absorption and secretion patterns, relying on time-course data rather than invasive intravenous insulin delivery [29]. Such approaches are particularly useful in early-stage clinical trials to assess insulin pharmacokinetics [29].

In a 2024 study with 21 healthy participants, researchers utilized these models to examine the effects of inhaled insulin (Technosphere® Insulin) during a standardized meal test [29]. The findings highlighted the models' ability to quantify how inhaled insulin influences endogenous insulin production, identifying a log-linear correlation between glycemic variability and endogenous insulin secretion [29]. This is especially relevant for type 2 diabetes patients, where residual endogenous insulin plays a significant role in total plasma insulin levels [29]. Inhaled insulin, a non-invasive alternative to injections, has shown benefits in easing patient burden and improving postprandial glucose control in both type 1 and type 2 diabetes [30]. By distinguishing between exogenous and endogenous insulin, these in silico models enable the design of individualized treatment plans, optimizing insulin dosing for improved glycemic outcomes [29].

EXPLORATION OF *IN SILICO* SENSORS

The physiological parameters related to diabetes are simulated and predicted with the help of *in silico* sensors using computational models. For digital healthcare technological advancements, computational tools help in the design and diagnosis of diabetes using *in silico* sensors. Traditionally, physical devices were required for trial as well as test purposes for the physiological measurements. But today, *in silico* sensors can simulate the complete process in a virtual and computational environment. These computational models help in the prediction of blood glucose levels, insulin dosages required, or even the design and development of treatments for various conditions of patients in a virtual environment. A basic structure of an *in silico* sensor is shown in Fig.(4).

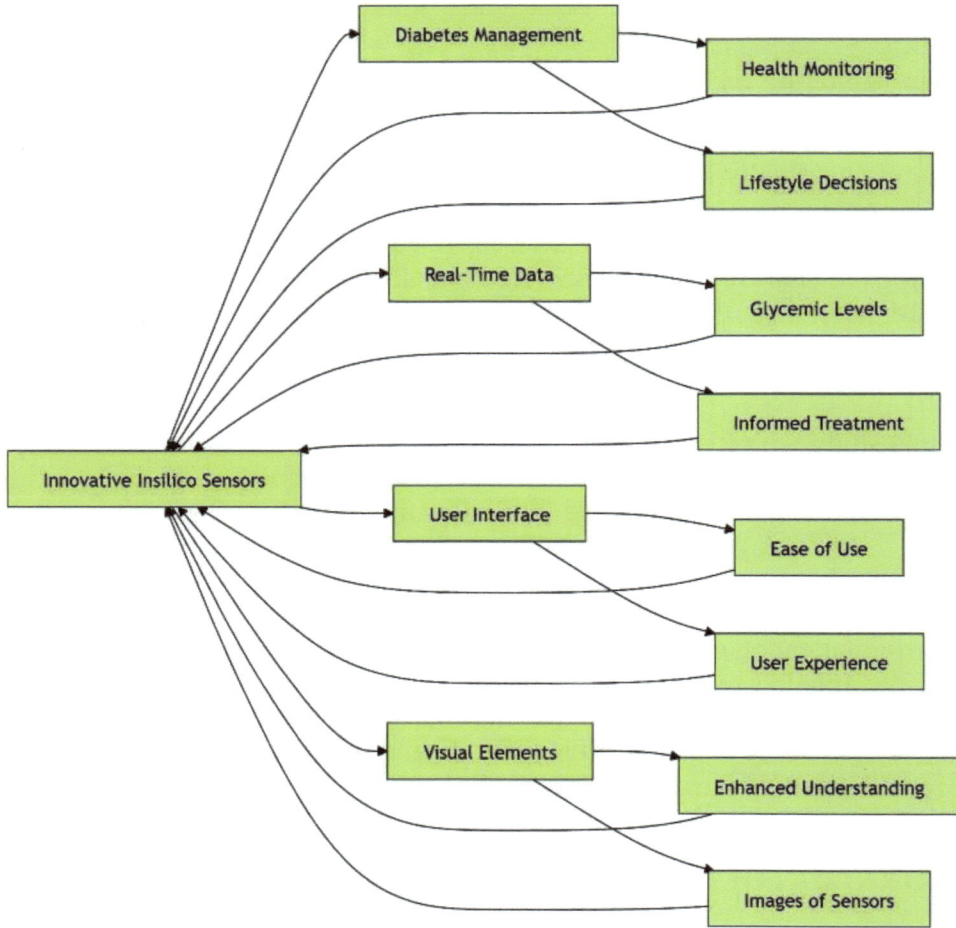

Fig. (4). Basic *in silico* sensor map.

In silico sensors are software-based tools that are designed using computer simulations and biological data. They are used to model complex biological processes with underlying mechanisms. Since *in vivo* and *in vitro* studies are costly and time-consuming, *in silico* modeling plays a very crucial role in the simulation and exploration of the dynamic interaction of several factors associated with metabolic disorders like diabetes. The model can simulate the metabolism of glucose, secretion of insulin, response to drugs, and various external inputs like food and physical activity.

The basic role of *in silico* sensors is covered in 3 steps:

Monitoring: Without any physical measurements required, *in silico* sensors can model the CGM and predict the glucose dynamics.

Prediction: *In silico* models can easily predict the trends of glucose based on the various patient conditions.

Personalized Medicine: *In silico* models are used to propose personalized medicine dosages and insulin requirements by simulating various conditions.

Optimization: These models can help optimize the delivery of insulin in the insulin pump as well as regulate CGM for an artificial pancreas device. Various mathematical computational models have been developed that can simulate the physiological processes associated with diabetes. Glucose-Insulin dynamics models includes Bergman minimal model, which describes a set of differential equations to relate glucose and insulin in the body, stochastic models, which mimic the effects of various factors like stress, exercise, and meal intake on glucose levels [31], Sedaghat model [32], which represents the insulin signaling pathways involved in glucose metabolism, and compartment models, which simulate the body by dividing it into various compartments like blood plasma, tissue, and interstitial fluid and establish the relationship between insulin and glucose [33, 34].

In silico models like one developed by Joshi *et al.* establish the relationship between medications like metformin, physical exercise, and natural herb oleuropein on the glucose levels in the body [35 - 38]. Additionally, Artificial Intelligence (AI) and Machine Learning (ML) can be used to boost the response of *in silico* sensors by providing various amounts of information received from physical wearable devices, insulin pumps, and CGMs for the prediction of glucose levels and hence manage diabetes.

Another technology that is in trend is the digital twin design of the real-world diabetic patient. This model virtually represents the insulin-glucose system, along with lifestyle, food habits, and various other relevant factors. Thus, with a digital twin, it becomes easier to predict future trends based on their physiological state. It helps in the identification of potential drug targets [39 - 41]. Further, virtual sensors based on algorithms are also in trend for the prediction of future glucose levels based on the inputs received as glucose, insulin, and physical workout data without being dependent on physical sensors. These algorithms, like Kalman filters and estimators, are integrated with CGM systems so that real-time data can be obtained.

In silico sensors can help in calibrating the CGMs by predicting the glucose profiles and thus provide personalized insulin therapy and medicine dosages. Also, the most important application of *in silico* sensors is the simulation carried out by pharmaceutical companies and healthcare researchers before conducting the real-world, costly, and time-consuming drug response clinical trials. Despite the advantages, the accuracy of *in silico* sensors depends largely on the availability of data and the dynamics of the detailed underlying mechanisms of signaling pathways, as simplified models may not predict the behavior accurately. Also, these models can only be used as a reference and may require regulations and validation approvals for any new medical advancements. Overall, *in silico* sensors play a significant role in the management of diabetes for the enhancement of patient outcomes.

CLOSED-LOOP CONTROL ALGORITHMS: TESTING AND EVALUATION

Closed-loop control, as the name suggests, closes the loop by using some feedback mechanism, such that the required state of the parameter is obtained in real time. For diabetes management, a closed-loop control system consists of a sensor, an error detector, a controller, and a process for which the control is needed. Control algorithms are used to manage insulin delivery for diabetic patients on the basis of glucose measurements. This algorithm is crucial as it manages the blood sugar levels by delivering the required amount of insulin by working as an artificial pancreas. These control algorithms are tested and evaluated for various input conditions, keeping in mind the external factors involved with diabetes care.

The main objective of closed-loop control is to maintain glucose homeostasis in the body. On the basis of CGM data, insulin delivery is adjusted. The closed-loop algorithm involved in glucose management is shown in Fig.(**5**).

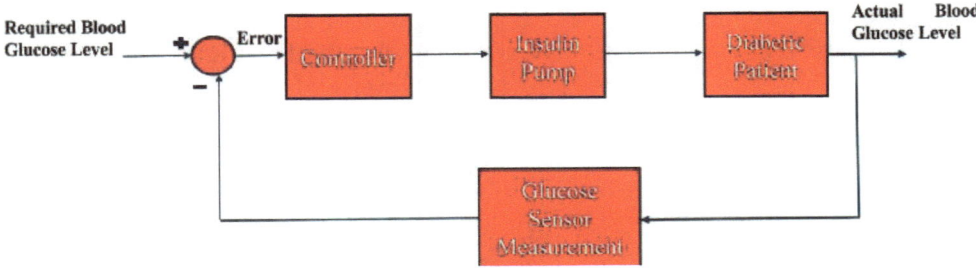

Fig. (5). Closed-loop algorithm for diabetes management.

As shown in the figure, the required blood glucose level is used as the set point for the system. In the feedback, a glucose sensor is placed, which measures the blood glucose level and sends this information to the controller, where, on the basis of the error generated, a predefined control algorithm generates a signal to the insulin pump to deliver the required amount of insulin to the diabetic patient. The loop stabilizes when the required amount of glucose is balanced in the body. CGM systems are used to continuously update the data of the glucose levels and hence adjust the rate of delivery by the insulin pump [42, 43].

Before implementation of the control loop, it is important that the loop is tested for safety and effectiveness, such that insulin delivery can take place appropriately on the basis of glucose fluctuations. The performance of the loop is evaluated and tested in a simulation environment first. Various *in silico* models are developed that integrate the insulin dynamics and glucose metabolism parameters so that the effect of medications, drug dosages, and control loop algorithms can be implemented and tested in virtual environments. It is used to estimate the response time of the control loop to variation in blood glucose levels and other factors like food intake, various intensities of physical activity, stress, illness, and obesity. Once the loop is tested in a virtual environment, hardware is introduced, and physical devices are then integrated with software to further simulate the glucose dynamics and send the simulated signals to insulin pumps for refined insulin delivery. The hardware is then evaluated for accuracy in insulin delivery [44 - 47].

Additionally, the loop is prepared for clinical trials to be carried out on actual patients in a controlled environment after being tested and assessed for hardware and software combinations. Trials are conducted on patients to evaluate the usefulness and efficiency of the control loop algorithms with the consent of various patient categories. This allows the glucose levels to be monitored using different insulin dosages based on control algorithms. It is crucial to remember that the control loop algorithm maintains the body's nominal blood glucose levels in order to ensure safety. Therefore, the loop's response time to inputs such as meals, exercise, and fasting is crucial [42 - 45, 48 - 50].

Also, with individuals' insulin sensitivities, it becomes difficult to predict the outcome of the loop. Thus, customization in the control loop algorithm is important to enhance personalized healthcare. Further, the response of the loop algorithm depends on the sensor delays and various other parameters, such as response time, which affects the outcomes of control loop algorithms in diabetes management. Following extensive testing, the algorithm is assessed by particular regulatory agencies before being made available for commerce in order to ensure patient safety [22, 23, 51]. Because it offers individualized automated healthcare, the control loop algorithm has the potential to improve the quality of life for those with diabetes, despite certain obstacles.

INSULIN PENS

An insulin pen is a simple, convenient, and accurate diabetes technological advancement. It is a medical injection device that delivers a prefilled amount of insulin into the innermost layer of the skin. It is an immensely popular form of diabetes therapy that helps manage the glucose levels in the body and is convenient to use in place of syringes. Simple and accurate delivery of insulin is possible with these insulin pens. For those patients who are taking multiple injections daily, insulin pens are a blessing. They come in various types, like some are pre-filled pens that have a specific dose of insulin, some are disposable pens, and some can be reused [52].

Pre-filled insulin pens have a cartridge that is filled with insulin, and one only needs to change the needle after each use. Once insulin is finished, it is either to be disposed of or reused, as mentioned on the pen. Lantus, Humalog, and NovoLog are some popular pre-filled insulin pens. In reusable insulin pens, one canreplace the cartridge once the insulin runs out, thus making them more effective. NovoPen and FlexPen are examples of reusable pens. Advancements have led to the development of smart insulin pens; they are equipped with smart technology that can connect the pens with mobile devices and hence create alerts on the basis of glucose levels and can also generate the trend. InPen and NovoPen with Bluetooth are some popular smart insulin pens. A sterile needle is attached to the pen filled with the required amount of insulin and injected into the body. Post injection, the needle is disposed of, and the insulin pen is stored at room temperature. NovoNordisk is one of the most popular brands of insulin pens. One such example is shown in (https://www.novonordisk.com/our-products/smar- -pens/novopen-6.html) (Fig.6).

Now, if we talk about the setting of the insulin dose, it is simple to adjust the dose of insulin with precision. They have disposable, small, and thin needles and hence provide a safe environment to the user. The insulin is visible from the outside, which makes it easier to refill the insulin cartridge when needed. Also, one particularly important feature of an insulin pen is the dose counter. It shows the number of insulin doses delivered. It is a compact device that is easy to carry and handle. Although the cost is higher, the accurate and easy-to-carry feature of insulin pens makes it a feasible option for diabetes management [53 - 57].

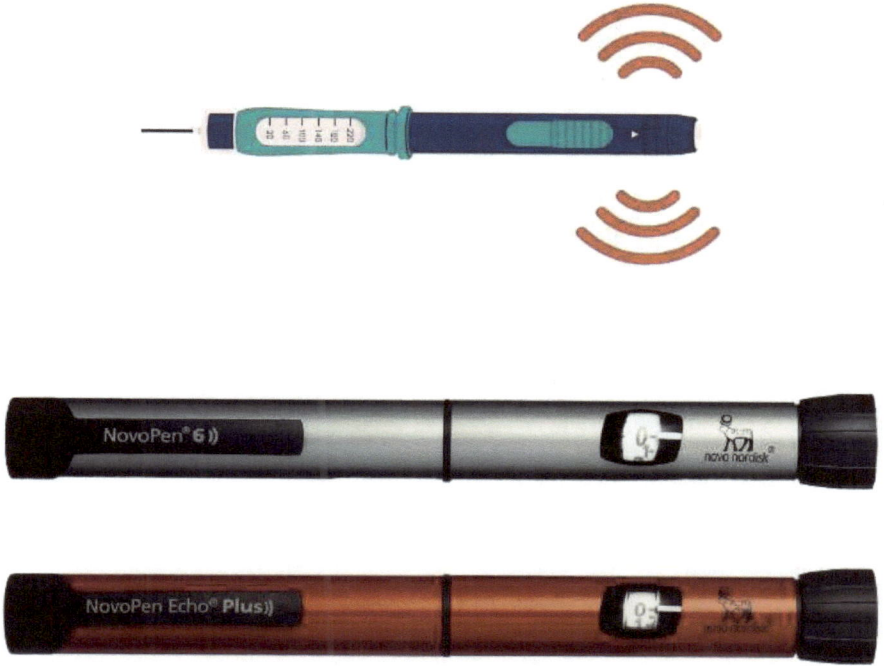

Fig. (6). Insulin pens.

CONCLUDING REMARKS

Diabetes management has greatly benefited from the use of technology such as insulin pumps, artificial pancreas systems, and Continuous Glucose Monitoring (CGM). These technologies offer automated, customized, and real-time insulin delivery to help diabetic patients maintain glucose homeostasis. Research on diabetes care has taken a new turn thanks to the use of *in silico* sensors and computational modeling. Personalized treatment is made possible by accurate and virtual models of the several biological pathways involved in diabetes. Furthermore, a potential automated insulin delivery system based on blood sugar changes is made possible by the use of strong closed-loop control algorithms. Additionally, smart insulin pens offer a dependable, portable, and easy-to-use approach for managing diabetes. Even though these technologies have a lot of promise, issues, including cost, data accuracy, and the requirement for regulatory monitoring, must be resolved to guarantee their success and broad adoption. Artificial Intelligence (AI) and Machine Learning (ML) will further improve diabetes care in the future. Diabetes care will be more automated and efficient thanks to this technology.

CONSENT FOR PUBLICATION

We hereby give consent for publication.

REFERENCES

[1]   Malek R, Davis SN. Novel methods of insulin replacement: The artificial pancreas and encapsulated islets. Rev Recent Clin Trials 2016; 11(2): 106-23.
        [http://dx.doi.org/10.2174/1574887111666151207112100] [PMID: 26638972]

[2]   Almurashi AM, Rodriguez E, Garg SK. Emerging diabetes technologies: Continuous glucose monitors/artificial pancreases. J Indian Inst Sci 2023; 103(1): 205-30.
        [http://dx.doi.org/10.1007/s41745-022-00348-3] [PMID: 37362851]

[3]   Allen N, Gupta A. Current diabetes technology: Striving for the artificial pancreas. Diagnostics (Basel) 2019; 9(1): 31.
        [http://dx.doi.org/10.3390/diagnostics9010031] [PMID: 30875898]

[4]   Shah NA, Levy CJ. Emerging technologies for the management of type 2 *Diabetes mellitus*. J Diabetes 2021; 13(9): 713-24.
        [http://dx.doi.org/10.1111/1753-0407.13188] [PMID: 33909352]

[5]   Moser EG, Morris AA, Garg SK. Emerging diabetes therapies and technologies. Diabetes Res Clin Pract 2012; 97(1): 16-26.
        [http://dx.doi.org/10.1016/j.diabres.2012.01.027] [PMID: 22381908]

[6]   Jiaojiao Y, Sun C, Wei Y, *et al.* Applying emerging technologies to improve diabetes treatment. Biomed Pharmacother 2018; 108: 1225-36.
        [http://dx.doi.org/10.1016/j.biopha.2018.09.155] [PMID: 30372824]

[7]   Kennedy ED, Oliver N. Emerging technologies for diabetes. Pract Diabetes 2017; 34(7): 240-4.
        [http://dx.doi.org/10.1002/pdi.2127]

[8]   Bailey TS, Walsh J, Stone JY. Emerging technologies for diabetes care. Diabetes Technol Ther 2018; 20(S2): S2-78-, S2-84.
        [http://dx.doi.org/10.1089/dia.2018.0115] [PMID: 29916738]

[9]   Brown C. 21st-Century Diabetes. NASN Sch Nurse 2016; 31(5): 254-6.
        [http://dx.doi.org/10.1177/1942602X16661198] [PMID: 27481481]

[10]   Klonoff DC, Ahn D, Drincic A. Continuous glucose monitoring: A review of the technology and clinical use. Diabetes Res Clin Pract 2017; 133: 178-92.
        [http://dx.doi.org/10.1016/j.diabres.2017.08.005] [PMID: 28965029]

[11]   Guerrero-Arroyo L, Faulds E, Perez-Guzman MC, Davis GM, Dungan K, Pasquel FJ. Continuous glucose monitoring in the intensive care unit. J Diabetes Sci Technol 2023; 17(3): 667-78.
        [http://dx.doi.org/10.1177/19322968231169522] [PMID: 37081830]

[12]   Avari P, Reddy M, Oliver N. Is it possible to constantly and accurately monitor blood sugar levels, in people with Type 1 diabetes, with a discrete device (non-invasive or invasive)? Diabet Med 2020; 37(4): 532-44.
        [http://dx.doi.org/10.1111/dme.13942] [PMID: 30803028]

[13]   Bailey TS. Clinical implications of accuracy measurements of continuous glucose sensors. Diabetes Technol Ther 2017; 19(S2): S-51-4.
        [http://dx.doi.org/10.1089/dia.2017.0050] [PMID: 28541134]

[14]   Martin CT, Criego AB, Carlson AL, Bergenstal RM. Advanced technology in the management of diabetes: Which comes first—continuous glucose monitor or insulin pump? Curr Diab Rep 2019; 19(8): 50.
        [http://dx.doi.org/10.1007/s11892-019-1177-7] [PMID: 31250124]

[15]   Carroll J, Heverly J, Phillip M, Battelino T, Garg S. International consensus of continuous glucose monitor use in pharmacological clinical trials in diabetes. Diabetes Technol Ther 2023; 25(4): 217-8.
[http://dx.doi.org/10.1089/dia.2023.0054] [PMID: 36730704]

[16]   Marks BE, Williams KM, Sherwood JS, Putman MS. Practical aspects of diabetes technology use: Continuous glucose monitors, insulin pumps, and automated insulin delivery systems. J Clin Transl Endocrinol 2022; 27: 100282.
[http://dx.doi.org/10.1016/j.jcte.2021.100282] [PMID: 34917483]

[17]   Schütz-Fuhrmann I, Rami-Merhar B, Fröhlich-Reiterer E, *et al.* Insulin pump therapy and continuous glucose monitoring. Wien Klin Wochenschr 2023; 135(S1) (Suppl. 1): 53-61.
[http://dx.doi.org/10.1007/s00508-023-02165-9] [PMID: 37101025]

[18]   McAdams B, Rizvi A. An overview of insulin pumps and glucose sensors for the generalist. J Clin Med 2016; 5(1): 5.
[http://dx.doi.org/10.3390/jcm5010005] [PMID: 26742082]

[19]   Faradji RN, De la Maza ES, Madrigal Sanromán JR. Insulin Pump Therapy. In: The diabetes textbook: Clinical principles, patient management and public health issues, second edition. 2023.
[http://dx.doi.org/10.1007/978-3-031-25519-9_38]

[20]   Hawlas H, Lewenstein K. The design of an insulin pump - preliminary requirements (a technical note). Polish Journal of Medical Physics And Engineering 2009; 15(1): 25-32.
[http://dx.doi.org/10.2478/v10013-009-0003-y]

[21]   Mughal IS, Patanè L, Caponetto R. A comprehensive review of models and nonlinear control strategies for blood glucose regulation in artificial pancreas. Annu Rev Contr 2024; 57: 100937.
[http://dx.doi.org/10.1016/j.arcontrol.2024.100937]

[22]   Nadia Ahmad NF, Nik Ghazali NN, Wong YH. Wearable patch delivery system for artificial pancreas health diagnostic-therapeutic application: A review. Biosens Bioelectron 2021; 189: 113384.
[http://dx.doi.org/10.1016/j.bios.2021.113384] [PMID: 34090154]

[23]   Quintal A, Messier V, Rabasa-Lhoret R, Racine E. A critical review and analysis of ethical issues associated with the artificial pancreas. Diabetes Metab 2019; 45(1): 1-10.
[http://dx.doi.org/10.1016/j.diabet.2018.04.003] [PMID: 29753624]

[24]   Peyser T, Dassau E, Breton M, Skyler JS. The artificial pancreas: Current status and future prospects in the management of diabetes. Ann N Y Acad Sci 2014; 1311(1): 102-23.
[http://dx.doi.org/10.1111/nyas.12431] [PMID: 24725149]

[25]   Nwokolo M, Hovorka R. The artificial pancreas and type 1 diabetes. J Clin Endocrinol Metab 2023; 108(7): 1614-23.
[http://dx.doi.org/10.1210/clinem/dgad068] [PMID: 36734145]

[26]   Lubinski T, Plotka B, Janik S, *et al.* Evaluation of a novel noninvasive blood glucose monitor based on mid-infrared quantum cascade laser technology and photothermal detection. In: Journal of Diabetes Science and Technology. 2020.
[http://dx.doi.org/10.1177/1932296820936634]

[27]   Breton MD, Kovatchev BP. One year real-world use of the control-iq advanced hybrid closed-loop technology. Diabetes Technol Ther 2021; 23(9): 601-8.
[http://dx.doi.org/10.1089/dia.2021.0097] [PMID: 33784196]

[28]   Zuijdwijk C, Courtney J, Mitsakakis N, *et al.* Control-IQ technology positively impacts patient reported outcome measures and glycemic control in youth with type 1 diabetes in a real-world setting. Pediatr Diabetes 2023.
[http://dx.doi.org/10.1155/2023/5106107]

[29]   Pinsker JE, Müller L, Constantin A, *et al.* Real-world patient-reported outcomes and glycemic results with initiation of control-IQ technology. Diabetes Technol Ther 2021; 23(2): 120-7.
[http://dx.doi.org/10.1089/dia.2020.0388] [PMID: 32846114]

[30]   Holt RIG, DeVries JH, Hess-Fischl A, *et al.* The management of type 1 diabetes in adults. A consensus report by the American Diabetes Association (ADA) and the European association for the study of diabetes (EASD). Diabetes Care 2021; 44(11): 2589-625.
[http://dx.doi.org/10.2337/dci21-0043] [PMID: 34593612]

[31]   Gallardo-Hernández AG, González-Olvera MA, Castellanos-Fuentes M, *et al.* Minimally-invasive and efficient method to accurately fit the bergman minimal model to diabetes type 2. Cell Mol Bioeng 2022; 15(3): 267-79.
[http://dx.doi.org/10.1007/s12195-022-00719-x] [PMID: 35611162]

[32]   Sedaghat AR, Sherman A, Quon MJ. A mathematical model of metabolic insulin signaling pathways. Am J Physiol Endocrinol Metab 2002; 283(5): E1084-101.
[http://dx.doi.org/10.1152/ajpendo.00571.2001] [PMID: 12376338]

[33]   Zhang Z, Zhan Q, Xie X. Numerical study on stochastic diabetes mellitus model with additive noise. J Diabetes Sci Technol 2019.
[http://dx.doi.org/10.1155/2019/5409180]

[34]   Duun-Henriksen AK, Schmidt S, Røge RM, *et al.* Model identification using stochastic differential equation grey-box models in diabetes. J Diabetes Sci Technol 2013; 7(2): 431-40.
[http://dx.doi.org/10.1177/193229681300700220] [PMID: 23567002]

[35]   Joshi DM, Patel J, Bhatt H. *In silico* study to quantify the effect of exercise on surface GLUT4 translocation in diabetes management. Netw Model Anal Health Inform Bioinform 2021; 10(1): 1.
[http://dx.doi.org/10.1007/s13721-020-00274-3]

[36]   Saiti K, Macaš M, Lhotská L, Štechová K, Pithová P. Ensemble methods in combination with compartment models for blood glucose level prediction in type 1 diabetes mellitus. Comput Methods Programs Biomed 2020; 196: 105628.
[http://dx.doi.org/10.1016/j.cmpb.2020.105628] [PMID: 32640369]

[37]   De Gaetano A, Hardy T, Beck B, *et al.* Mathematical models of diabetes progression. Am J Physiol Endocrinol Metab 2008; 295(6): E1462-79.
[http://dx.doi.org/10.1152/ajpendo.90444.2008] [PMID: 18780774]

[38]   Kwaghkor LM, Mohammed A, Nyamtswam EV. A MATHEMATICAL MODEL FOR DIABETES MANAGEMENT. FUDMA JOURNAL OF SCIENCES 2022; 6(5): 36-40.
[http://dx.doi.org/10.33003/fjs-2022-0605-1091]

[39]   Zhang Y, Qin G, Aguilar B, *et al.* A framework towards digital twins for type 2 diabetes. Frontiers in Digital Health 2024; 6: 1336050.
[http://dx.doi.org/10.3389/fdgth.2024.1336050] [PMID: 38343907]

[40]   Chu Y, Li S, Tang J, Wu H. The potential of the Medical Digital Twin in diabetes management: a review. Front Med (Lausanne) 2023; 10: 1178912.
[http://dx.doi.org/10.3389/fmed.2023.1178912] [PMID: 37547605]

[41]   Thamotharan P, Srinivasan S, Kesavadev J, *et al.* Human digital twin for personalized elderly type 2 diabetes management. J Clin Med 2023; 12(6): 2094.
[http://dx.doi.org/10.3390/jcm12062094] [PMID: 36983097]

[42]   Kovatchev B. Automated closed-loop control of diabetes: The artificial pancreas. Bioelectron Med 2018; 4(1): 14.
[http://dx.doi.org/10.1186/s42234-018-0015-6] [PMID: 32232090]

[43]   Nimri R, Phillip M, Clements MA, Kovatchev B. Closed-loop control, artificial intelligence–based decision-support systems, and data science. Diabetes Technol Ther 2024; 26(S1): S-68-89.
[http://dx.doi.org/10.1089/dia.2024.2505] [PMID: 38441444]

[44]   Cobelli C, Pacini G, Ruggeri A, *et al.* Algorithms for closed-loop glucose control (artificial pancreas) in diabetes - a novel noninvasive approach for their evaluation based on mathematical modeling 1982.
[http://dx.doi.org/10.1016/S1474-6670(17)64026-6]

[45]   Estremera E, Beneyto A, Cabrera A, Contreras I, Vehí J. Intermittent closed-loop blood glucose control for people with type 1 diabetes on multiple daily injections. Comput Methods Programs Biomed 2023; 236: 107568.
[http://dx.doi.org/10.1016/j.cmpb.2023.107568] [PMID: 37137221]

[46]   El Youssef J, Castle J, Ward WK. A review of closed-loop algorithms for glycemic control in the treatment of type 1 diabetes. Algorithms 2009; 2(1): 518-32.
[http://dx.doi.org/10.3390/a2010518]

[47]   Chen J, Cao K, Sun Y, *et al.* Continuous drug infusion for diabetes therapy: A closed-loop control system design. Eurasip J Wirel Commun Netw 2008.
[http://dx.doi.org/10.1155/2008/495185]

[48]   Chassin LJ, Wilinska ME, Hovorka R. Evaluation of glucose controllers in virtual environment: methodology and sample application. Artif Intell Med 2004; 32(3): 171-81.
[http://dx.doi.org/10.1016/j.artmed.2004.02.006] [PMID: 15531149]

[49]   Percival MW, Zisser H, Jovanovič L, Doyle FJ III. Closed-loop control and advisory mode evaluation of an artificial pancreatic β cell: Use of proportional-integral-derivative equivalent model-based controllers. J Diabetes Sci Technol 2008; 2(4): 636-44.
[http://dx.doi.org/10.1177/193229680800200415] [PMID: 19885240]

[50]   Wilinska ME, Chassin LJ, Acerini CL, Allen JM, Dunger DB, Hovorka R. Simulation environment to evaluate closed-loop insulin delivery systems in type 1 diabetes. J Diabetes Sci Technol 2010; 4(1): 132-44.
[http://dx.doi.org/10.1177/193229681000400117] [PMID: 20167177]

[51]   Dassau E, Jimenez ND, Zisser HC, Jovanovic L, Doyle FJ. The artificial pancreas system, a comprehensive system for the clinical evaluation of control algorithms. Diabetes Technol Ther 2011; 13(2): 179.

[52]   Kroon L. Overview of insulin delivery pen devices. J Am Pharm Assoc (Wash DC) 2009; 49(5): e118-31.
[http://dx.doi.org/10.1331/JAPhA.2009.08125] [PMID: 19692314]

[53]   Lingen K, Pikounis T, Bellini N, Isaacs D. Advantages and disadvantages of connected insulin pens in diabetes management. Endocr Connect 2023; 12(11): e230108.
[http://dx.doi.org/10.1530/EC-23-0108] [PMID: 37610002]

[54]   Heinemann L, Schnell O, Gehr B, Schloot NC, Görgens SW, Görgen C. Digital diabetes management: A literature review of smart insulin pens. J Diabetes Sci Technol 2022; 16(3): 587-95.
[http://dx.doi.org/10.1177/1932296820983863] [PMID: 33430644]

[55]   Tosun B, Cinar FI, Topcu Z, *et al.* Do patients with diabetes use the insulin pen properly? Afr Health Sci 2019; 19(1): 1628-37.
[http://dx.doi.org/10.4314/ahs.v19i1.38] [PMID: 31148992]

[56]   Cranston I, Jamdade V, Liao B, Newson RS. Clinical, economic, and patient-reported benefits of connected insulin pen systems: A systematic literature review. Adv Ther 2023; 40(5): 2015-37.
[http://dx.doi.org/10.1007/s12325-023-02478-1] [PMID: 36928495]

[57]   Rubin RR, Peyrot M. Factors affecting use of insulin pens by patients with type 2 diabetes. Diabetes Care 2008; 31(3): 430-2.
[http://dx.doi.org/10.2337/dc07-1899] [PMID: 18039802]

CHAPTER 4

In Silico **Modeling and Simulation Approaches**

Abstract: Computational advancements have emerged in recent years, and *in silico* modeling has been introduced as a powerful tool in diabetes management. Various biotechnological tools, such as MATLAB, Simulink, COPASI, Cell Designer, and Multiphysics, have enhanced the understanding of complex biological phenomena involved in the insulin-glucose pathway. This chapter emphasizes the utilization of *biotechnological* tools in simulating the dynamics of glucose regulation and artificial pancreas control systems. The kinetics of insulin through PKPD parameters-based models that define the insulin action, absorption variability, and dynamics of glucose regulation are explored. A case study on the modeling of insulin infusion pumps that control insulin release and, as a result, preserve glucose levels is thoroughly examined. Naturopathy is taken into consideration in another case study that examines the effects of alternative therapy on diabetes. Furthermore, data-driven diabetes management models are analyzed, and their potential to forecast tailored healthcare that can enhance therapeutic outcomes in diabetes care is explored.

Keywords: Case study, Diabetes, *In silico*, Insulin pump, PKPD, Simulation.

INTRODUCTION

Diabetes mellitus, one of the most troubling and complex disorders on the globe, is caused by uncontrolled hyperglycemia. It is a chronic metabolic disorder. Insulin secretion, glucose regulation, and cellular metabolism all directly correlate with the causes of diabetes. The traditional approach to diabetes treatment is based on clinical evaluation, medication, and lifestyle modification. With improved comprehension of the disease, sharper and more directed treatment options need to be deployed. Therefore, advanced technology and AI algorithms are being deployed for handling diabetes more easily and developing innovations for treatment on a higher level. *In silico* approaches are being adapted for diabetes amelioration, which is baffling for an average human being.

The comprehension of diabetes and its processes on a biological level, especially the control of blood sugar, has grown tremendously with the sharp advancement of computer power and biotechnology tools. *In silico* models can increase our comprehension of insulin delivery, glucose balance, and other forms of

Darshna M. Joshi, Hardik Bhatt & Himanshu K. Patel

treatment offered. With this in mind, advanced simulation tools have emerged, such as MATLAB, Simulink, CoPASI, Cell Designer, Multiphysics, which help design and simulate unparalleled models interfacing the insulin-glucose system.

Such tools assist scientists in building and assessing static models that consider the impact of insulin infusion, diet, exercise, and other treatments on blood sugar control. The combination of clinical and experimental data with the *in silico* model has paved the way for additional possibilities to formulate and refine treatment plans. One of the ways in which biomedical models have improved diabetes care is through the creation of an artificial pancreas system, which integrates continuous glucose monitoring and insulin infusion pumping. These models also help in the optimization of insulin dosing by simulating insulin delivery, insulin action, and glucose consumption, which will ultimately improve insulin dosing accuracy, minimize the challenges of hypoglycemia, and improve overall glucose management.

This chapter presents a study on the application of computational modeling, simulation, and analysis of insulin-dependent diabetes mellitus, with particular attention to the technological instruments used during the simulation of the insulin-glucose relationship and control of the artificial pancreas. It also covers clinical studies on insulin infusion pumps and case studies of patients who received alternative therapy with insulin, showing how model-driven approaches can be used for developing tailored therapies. These methods help the patients by offering new forms of healthcare that can be more personalized and useful, as well as making it simpler to address the core reasons for diabetes.

UTILIZATION OF BIOTECHNOLOGICAL TOOLS: MATLAB, SIMULINK, COPASI, CELL DESIGNER, MULTIPHYSICS

Biotechnological tools are used for the analysis of various biological disease mechanisms. Diabetes is a metabolic disorder that is caused by disruptions in the underlying mechanisms. These mechanisms have yet to be fully revealed, and hence, it is difficult to analyze the disease mechanism directly through *in vivo* or *in vitro* studies. Here comes the role of biotechnological tools, which are used to successfully design and develop the mechanism of various diseases, and one can easily analyze the impact of various factors on the model outcome. Even variations in biological parameters with an infinite range of combinations are possible to be tested with an *in silico* model. This section will discuss various biotechnological tools like MATLAB, Simulink, Copasi, Cell Designer, and Multiphysics, with a focus on the simulation and analysis of diabetes mechanisms. Various features available with the biotechnological tools are shown in Table **1** [1 - 4].

Table 1. Biotechnological tools and their features [1–4].

Software	Matlab	Copasi	Cell Designer	Comsol Multiphysics
Features	Simulink	Model Building and Editing	Graphical Modeling Interface	Chemical Reaction Engineering Module
	SimBiology	Simulation and Time-course Analysis	Rule-Based Modeling	Biological Reaction Engineering Module
	Statistics and Machine Learning Toolbox	Parameter Estimation	Pathway Visualization	Transport of Diluted Species Module
	Deep Learning Toolbox	Optimization	s BML (Systems Biology Markup Language) Export and Import	Heat Transfer Module
	Signal Processing Toolbox	Sensitivity Analysis	Simulation (Deterministic and Stochastic)	Electromagnetic Module
	Optimization Toolbox	Stochastic Simulation (SSA)	Qualitative Simulation	Microfluidics Module
	Control System Toolbox	Flux Balance Analysis (FBA)	Parameter Estimation	Live Link for MA TLAB
	Bioinformatics Toolbox	Bifurcation Analysis	Sensitivity Analysis	Multibody Dynamics Module
	Image Processing Toolbox	Stoichiometric Analysis	Bifurcation Analysis	Optimization Module
	Curve Fitting Toolbox	Data Fitting	Model Validation	Human Models (Customizable Tissue and Organ Models
	Time Series Toolbox	Pathway Analysis	Model Libraries	Diabetes Simulation, Artificial Pancreas Systems
	Network Toolbox (now part of the Deep Learning)	Monte Carlo Simulation	Time-course Simulation	Coupled Multiphysics Simulation
	Data Acquisition Toolbox	Control Analysis	Automatic Diagram Layout	Flow and Reaction in Porous Media
	Mapping Toolbox	Network Visualization	Network Topology Analysis	Fluid-Structure Interaction
	Instrument Control Toolbox	Import and Export (SBML, SED-ML, *etc.*)	Gene regulatory network modeling	Bioheat Transfer
	Healthcare Analytics Toolbox	Metabolic Control Analysis (MCA)	Metabolic Network Modeling	Tissue Engineering and Growth Models

Software	Matlab	Copasi	Cell Designer	Comsol Multiphysics
Features	System Identification Toolbox	Genetic Algorithm for Optimization	Control and Feedback Analysis	System Design and Control (Model-Based Design)
		Time-Series Data Analysis	Multi-compartment Modeline	
		Parameter Scanning	Parameter Scanning	
		Model Comparison and Validation	Plugin Support (*e.g.*, Copasi, GINsim, etc.)	

A simulation model of the glucose-insulin dynamic mechanism helps to test and evaluate the control algorithms with respect to the glucose levels in response to insulin delivery with various factors, including stress, physical activity, and meals. MATLAB (**MATrix LABoratory**) and Simulink are widely used to design disease-based models and analyze the complex biological mechanisms. Chiara *et al*. [5] introduced a software for the meal Glucose-insulin Model (GIM) in MATLAB version 7.0.1. The model simulates the function of the liver, GI tract, muscle adipose tissue, and beta cells of the pancreas. Insulin kinetics are simulated in the model with the help of a set of mathematical equations defining each compartment. When the user runs the model, a pop-up box is displayed, and one needs to select the status of the patient, whether Type 1 Diabetic, Type 2 Diabetic, or Normal. Once the required status of the patient is selected, a new window opens asking for the meal ingestion time. With all the details inputted, graphical representations of the glucose and insulin concentrations, glucose production, and insulin secretion are available to the user. The same model is also implemented using Simulink of MATLAB, where one can test the closed-loop control algorithms for the artificial pancreas to predict the dose of insulin for glucose management. Although the model is very useful, the physiological knowledge of the parameters is extremely crucial for the accuracy of the model output.

Muhammad Mufti *et al*. [6] developed a model to showcase the dynamic interaction between glucose and insulin for type 1 diabetic subjects. An extended version of the Bergman minimal model was used, and using state-space equations, the Simulink model was developed for the open-loop as well as the closed-loop method. The mathematical model gave us a deep insight into the choice of appropriate controller configuration for the development of closed-loop control algorithms for glucose insulin management in diabetes. Another model that is interesting to discuss here is the model developed by Hanane *et al*. [7]. An optimal control theory is applied to Bergman's minimal model, and a solution is obtained using MATLAB, for both with-control and without-control numerical equations of the model. The output shows a reduction in the glycemic conditions of the subject.

Another model that concerns the optimization approach of MATLAB's SimBiology tool is the one developed by Joshi *et al.* [8, 9]. The model is the only model available so far to simulate the effect of metformin, oleuropein herbs, and physical exercise of various intensities on glucose levels in T2D conditions. Sobol sensitivity analysis is a global sensitivity analysis method used to determine how the uncertainty in the output of a model can be attributed to different input variables, including their interactions. It decomposes the variance of the model output into fractions that can be attributed to inputs or combinations of inputs. Sobol sensitivity analysis is also carried out to obtain the potential drug targets, which are helpful in drug discovery for the pharmaceutical industries. Further, an imitation of the pancreas was developed mathematically by Jameel *et al.* [10]. Using this model, a closed-loop control system that regulates and manages the blood glucose-insulin has been designed using MATLAB/Simulink. Based on various parameters, simulations were carried out for diabetes management analysis using this model. Hence, it is very clear that MATLAB/Simulink plays a major role in the analysis of various dynamic conditions of the model with diabetes [6, 7, 10 - 13].

MATLAB is an advanced tool that can easily process and analyze complex biological data. It can perform statistical analysis as well as build and train models using AI and ML techniques. Various complex modeling equations can easily be solved using MATLAB, which is very crucial for understanding biological mechanisms. Optimization tools can be used in MATLAB that can provide the optimum dosage data for various metabolic disorders. Various tools and applications like Simulink and SimBiology are available in the MATLAB environment, which can analyze complex biological networks of diabetes, along with the effects of various allopathic and alternative therapies on diabetes management. Biomedical health data analysis can be carried out using a bioinformatics toolbox.

Simulink, which is another extension of MATLAB, is a block-based tool. Users can pick and place blocks and build the required model. Dynamic simulations are carried out, and the effect of variations in parameters over time can be logged and observed using graphs. The best advantage of Simulink is the integration of biological models and control systems with the real hardware systems [1, 10, 13 - 18]. This can help pharmacological researchers to test medicines, as well as industries to test wearable medical devices. Hence, MATLAB and Simulink are versatile tools that have revolutionized the biotechnological world.

COPASI is another powerful biotechnological tool that can simulate and perform various interactive analyses on biological data. The biochemical interactions between glucose and insulin can be simulated using the tool. Complex metabolic pathways can be analyzed, and estimation of parameters, sensitivity analysis, and bifurcation analysis can be carried out using this software tool. The study of metabolic networks in insulin signaling pathways, which is known as Flux Balance Analysis (FBA), is done with COPASI. Ultimately, the uncertainty and variability in the data of the model can be studied in detail with Monte Carlo simulations performed using the software [2, 19 - 22].

Yoke *et al.*, in a recent article, carried out the *in silico* identification of metabolites that contribute to the development of T2DM. An interesting approach is applied, where the key intermediates of the insulin signaling pathways, viz. PKB/Akt, PKC-ζ, and GLUT4 were analyzed using the software COPASI. Disruptions in these key parameters were introduced in the model, and *in silico* results were obtained to identify the potential targets for diabetic drugs. Another model developed by Deepa *et al.* [23] showed how glucose-stimulated insulin secretion takes place and how ATP/ADP factors affect the insulin secretion in the pancreas. Janis *et al.* further explored the impact of metformin transport rates on humans. Metformin is one of the most prescribed drugs for diabetes treatment. The model to simulate the effect of metformin transport rate was developed in COPASI. The model could successfully simulate the distribution dynamics of metformin between red blood cells and plasma for diabetes management [24]. COPASI thus provides a tool that can help basic researchers in identifying potential drug targets by performing sensitivity analysis, optimization, and stochastic simulations.

Cell Designer is an open-source biochemical network simulator that is used for developing various metabolic pathways. Joshi *et al.* developed and analyzed insulin signaling pathways with the effect of exercise, metformin, and medicinal herbs using Cell Designer [8, 9, 25, 26]. It is the only model available that possesses the ability to model the signaling pathways with the effects of alternative therapies. This *in silico* model utilized the Cell Designer software to design the pathways and then integrated with COPASI and Systems Biology Workbench (SBW) available with it. The model from Cell Designer can be stored as Systems Biology Markup Language (SBML) and can be exported or imported to/from MATLAB as well as COPASI and other plugins for further processing. Thus, for analyzing the complex biological pathways, Cell Designer holds a promising role as it is available for free with the advantage of integration with various software. Along with rule-based modeling, time course simulation can be very easily performed using Cell Designer, and plugins' support is even more commendable [3, 27, 28].

Instead of carrying out the costly and time-consuming *in vivo* or *in vitro* analysis, Cell Designer helps in the analysis of the underlying mechanisms of drug-receptor interactions in diabetes. Metabolic insulin signaling pathways were analyzed by Eric *et al.* [29]. They performed sensitivity analysis by introducing perturbations in the pathway and examined the effect to identify the potential targets for diabetes management. The model proposed by Sedaghat *et al.* [30] was utilized as a reference to perform sensitivity analysis.

Now, an ultimately different kind of biotechnological tool is COMSOL Multiphysics. It is used for the analysis of complex biological processes of diabetes research that incorporates the heat and mass transfer effects by performing electrochemical analysis. This tool offers specialized modules for carrying out the implementation of biological reactions and metabolic effects, as well as the dynamics of fluids, their interactions, and the heat transfer associated with the biochemical reactions carried out in the pathways. Systems like insulin secretion in the pancreas, the mechanism of glucose transporters, as well as the binding of drugs and receptors, all involve chemical reactions. These interactions play a crucial role in analyzing what is possible with tools like Multiphysics.

Peter *et al.* [4] developed an exploratory model of glucose-insulin dynamics using COMSOL. With COMSOL Multiphysics, the complex equations of insulin secretion and the glucose consumption kinetics can be easily described. The results of the model can help researchers tune and model the artificial pancreas as the dynamics are analyzed. Pareek *et al.* [31] developed a mathematical model of the glucose-sensitive hydrogel to analyze the swelling behaviors observed in patients with diabetes. This can help design the drug delivery systems for diabetic patients in a better way that can control swelling and other associated disorders.

Marra *et al.* is another researcher who used COMSOL Multiphysics [32] for the development of an integrated sensor design for glucose monitoring. By analyzing the chemical, electrical, and biological interactions within these systems, one can optimize the design and measurement techniques for developing diabetes sensors.

The efficient implementation of advances in technology is made possible using biotechnological techniques to evaluate the intricate biological networks involved in diabetes research. This strategy encourages the creation of new medications and complementary therapies for the worldwide treatment of diabetes.

INSULIN ACTION AND ABSORPTION VARIABILITY: *IN SILICO* MODELING

Various biotechnological tools are utilized for the *in silico* modeling of glucose metabolism. However, for diabetes management, the variation in insulin absorption in individuals plays a vital role. This section discusses the *in silico* modeling of insulin action and absorption variability. Such models are important to study the effect of insulin absorption variation in different individuals with diabetes. These models help in the incorporation of various factors like pharmacological, biological, kinetic, and physiological. Hence, the healthcare researchers can estimate the behavior of insulin in the body in the presence of different environmental conditions, undergoing various treatments.

The ADME (Absorption, Distribution, Metabolism, and Excretion) model is the most popular one that explains how a drug moves and gets processed in the body. Insulin is a crucial anabolic hormone generated by the pancreas and is responsible for the metabolism of carbohydrates and the generation of ATP. In the adipose muscles, this hormone converts glucose into lactate and vice versa in the liver. Also, the suppression of glucose production and glycogen synthesis is carried out by insulin in the liver. It thus directs the metabolism of the fuel sources in the body [33].

In silico modeling approaches have made the quantitative decision faster through various pharmacokinetic–pharmacodynamic (PKPD) models as well as newly available preclinical and clinical data. This provides an accurate prediction regarding the response of insulin in individuals. The insulin pharmacokinetics model simulates how insulin is absorbed, distributed, metabolized, and excreted from the body. Variability is observed based on factors such as the site of injection of insulin, its formulation, and the characteristics of individual diabetic patients. The insulin pharmacodynamics model simulates the effects of insulin on glucose metabolism and insulin resistance in the body. The variation in insulin sensitivity with varying levels of glucose can be easily understood with such models. The body mass index is influenced by several individual factors, such as age, weight, genetics, and food habits [34 - 42].

Physical activity has a significant impact on insulin action and absorption. The glucose-insulin model of dynamics helps predict the glucose levels and insulin resistance variation over time. With individual variations, one can even provide personalized treatment for diabetes using these models. As discussed in the previous chapter, the integration of advanced technologies with simulations provides a fruitful approach to diabetes management. An artificial pancreas is one such system in which the control algorithm can be managed based on the *in silico* model's outcomes, and this can be integrated with the insulin pumps to manage glucose levels. Models, such as drugs like metformin, herbs like Oleuropein, and physical activity, are available that help enhance GLUT4 (glucose transporter 4) translocation and manage diabetes [43 - 46].

Similar insulin dosages have different effects on metabolism, as demonstrated by Lutz *et al.* [47]. Therefore, the model must consider the PKPD kinetics variables. The effect and absorption of insulin molecules are significantly influenced by the local blood flow in the subcutaneous tissue. Insulin preparation variables such as volume and concentration, injection site changes such as insulin depths, and the impact of internal and external environmental factors such as age, massage, smoking, exercise, and temperature are the main factors that affect the variability of insulin absorption.

A highly intriguing pedagogical evaluation of the application of PKPD concepts to insulin therapy in type 2 diabetes was conducted by Arnolds *et al.* [48]. After a thorough examination of the literature, it was determined that PD parameters are more important for insulin therapy than PK parameters. There was a discussion about PK's limitations over PD parameters. The best way to determine insulin PD was described, along with the glucose-clamp methodology. The results were compared with the available clinical trial data, and the optimal basal insulin dosage was investigated. Algorithms for conducting clinical trials for insulin therapy have been developed with the assistance of the review.

Senshang Lin *et al.* developed an *in silico* model of PKPD parameters in comparison to the effect-compartment link model [49]. Healthy minipigs received a regular dosage of human insulin, and their blood glucose levels were continuously tracked. Indirect PD models were shown to be more suitable than effect-compartment link models after the data was fitted to PKPD models to analyze the blood glucose and plasma insulin profiles.

Additionally, using PKPD data, Kristine *et al.* presented an *in silico* model to investigate the kinetics of the glucose-insulin response. As a reference model, they employed the Hovorka model. To treat diabetes, PKPD models were selected for additional investigation based on experimental data of glucose-insulin response. Robust closed-loop algorithms for an artificial pancreas that can better control diabetes can be developed with the use of such simulations [50].

Another interesting model was presented by Edoardo *et al.* [51]. Based on subject variability, a model was created that could offer a more thorough knowledge of the insulin absorption process. This model can aid in the construction of open-loop or closed-loop algorithms that offer diabetic patients individualized treatment plans. A pictorial representation of the modeling approach used is shown in Fig.(**1**). It is evident from this that *in silico* models offer a valid and efficient means of analyzing insulin absorption and variability in diabetic individuals and, consequently, forecasting individualized treatment plans to improve lifestyles globally.

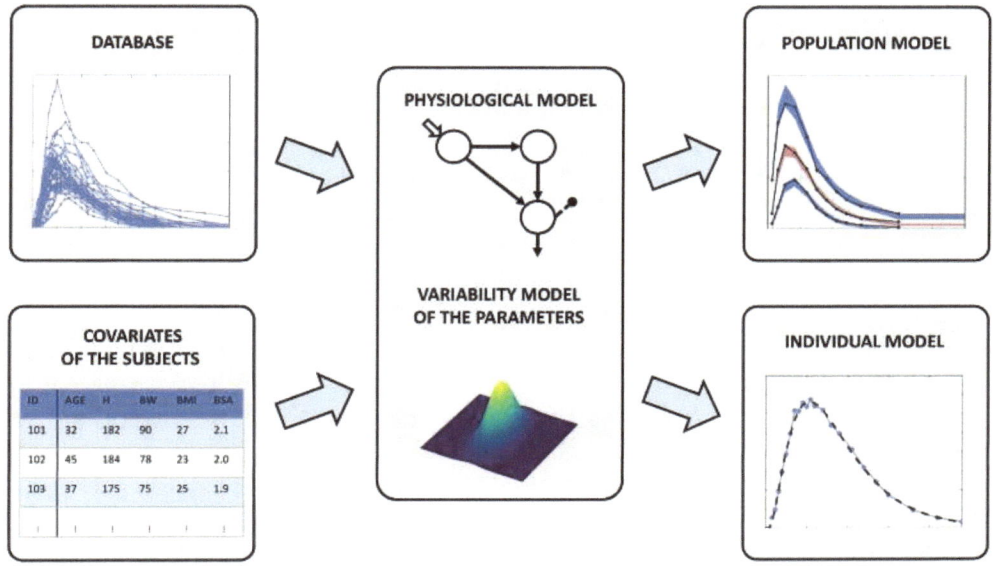

Fig. (1). Insulin absorption model.

CASE STUDY ON INSULIN INFUSION PUMP: *IN SILICO* MODELING

In silico modeling for insulin infusion pumps plays a crucial role in the management of diabetes. These models help predict the algorithm structure and hence guide the delivery of insulin, thereby maintaining the glucose levels based on real-time measurement data. Here, we have presented a case study of an insulin infusion pump [51] for the better understanding of the insulin infusion pump system in type 1 diabetes patients.

Objective: Create a personalized *in silico* model for insulin infusion pumps.

Approach:

- To create an insulin infusion pump, control software design for individualized treatment was used. The structure controls blood glucose levels by simulating the pancreatic function in the body. Blood glucose regulation is influenced by user factors such as meal intake, digestive speed, and the efficiency of the body's metabolism. Therefore, there is a complicated link between insulin injection therapy and glucose levels. To adjust the insulin dosage as needed, the insulin infusion pump's control system algorithm must be reliable. One system that is essential to safety is the control system. The body's glucose homeostasis will be disrupted if the system is unable to inject the appropriate amount of insulin, which can have major health effects.

- **Stakeholder:** Diabetic patients, healthcare practitioners, caretakers, insulin pump making industries, pharmaceutical companies, and nurses.
- **Description**
  1. A sensor that is placed in the patient's body is used by the control system to measure the glucose level.
  2. The controller with the desired logic program compares consecutive glucose level readings, and if the level increases, insulin pumps are instructed to release insulin to bring the levels back into balance. The setpoint is maintained so that the user's blood sugar levels remain within a healthy range.
  3. If the device is wirelessly connected, alerts or notifications are sent to the user or other stakeholders if insulin delivery issues occur. When a patient's characteristics vary significantly over time, the likelihood of an error increases.
  4. When making decisions, the model considers individual data such as body mass index, dietary patterns, and physical exercise regimens.
  5. The system is modified in real time to control the body's blood glucose levels.

The presented *in silico* model case study shows that meal intake, exercise, and various characteristics of diabetic individuals are simulated and provides an insulin input to maintain the glucose levels in the body. The architecture is shown in Fig.**2** and Fig.**3.** It reveals that the simulation of an insulin infusion pump can help better manage diabetes by taking care of all the factors.

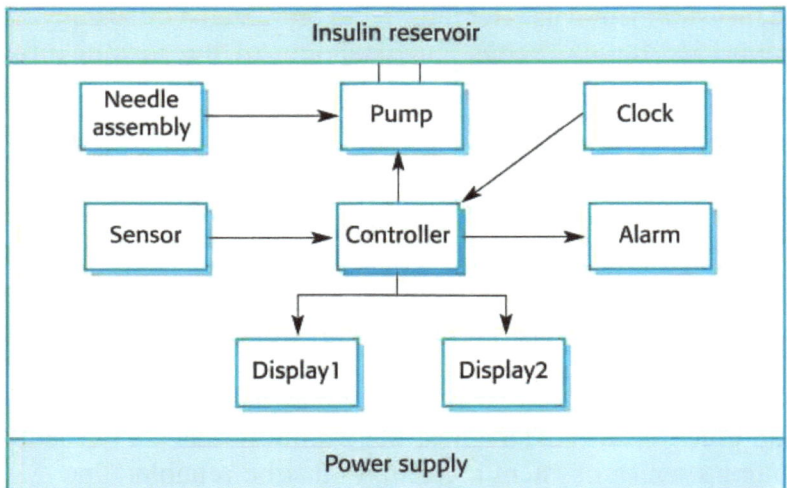

Fig. (2). Insulin pump architecture (Hardware).

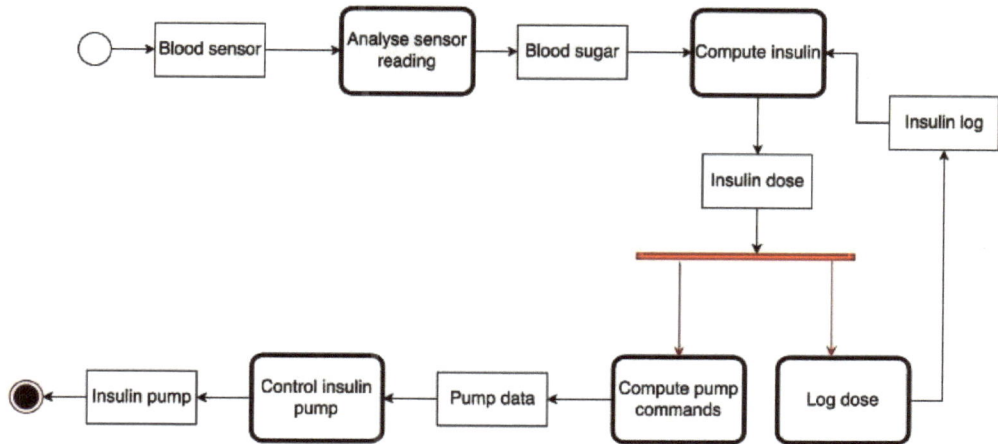

Fig. (3). Insulin pump's activity diagram.

CASE STUDY ON THE MODELING IMPACT OF ALTERNATIVE THERAPIES IN DIABETES MANAGEMENT

Diabetes is a metabolic disorder that has found no complete cure to date. However, allopathic medicines are recommended for the management of diabetes. The long-term complications and side effects of these allopathic drugs are a matter of worry. Alternative therapies like exercise, natural herbs, yoga, and acupuncture will play a vital role in overcoming complications in the future. *In silico* models that explore the effect of exercise and oleuropein, a natural herb, on glucose regulation in type 2 diabetes have been developed and analyzed [8, 25]. A case study [51] on modeling the impact of alternative therapy for diabetes management is presented here.

With an emphasis on the effects of dietary modifications, lifestyle adjustments, and therapeutic techniques on blood sugar regulation, weight management, and general health, this case study investigates the use of naturopathy and alternative therapies [51]:

- **Patient Profile**
  - **Age**: 48 years
  - **Weight**: 75 kg
  - **Diagnosis**: Type 2 Diabetes Mellitus (T2DM)
  - **Symptoms**: Leg pain, knee pain, back pain, weakness, improper digestion, constipation, and classic diabetes symptoms (e.g., increased thirst, hunger, frequent urination).

- **Past Medical History**: Hypertension, Type 2 diabetes mellitus (diagnosed), currently on diabetic medications (Metformin) and antihypertensive therapy (Lisinopril and Clonidine).

- **Initial Investigational Reports**
  - **Blood Pressure (BP)**: 140/95 mmHg
  - **Fasting Blood Sugar (BSL-F)**: 120 mg/dL
  - **Postprandial Blood Sugar (PP)**: 160 mg/dL (after taking diabetic tablet)
  - **HBA1C**: 8.6%

According to these initial values, the patient is experiencing hypertension and poor blood sugar management, both of which are prevalent in Type 2 diabetes.

- **Naturopathy Treatment Approach**

In addition to standard diabetic drugs, the patient's treatment regimen included dietary strategies and lifestyle changes. Among the naturopathic treatments were:

1. Yoga, Pranayama, and Walking
2. Dietary Changes
3. Lifestyle Modifications
4. Results After One Month of Therapy [51].

Following the naturopathy treatment plan for the first month, the following findings were noted:

- Blood pressure dropped from 140/95 mmHg to 138/90 mmHg.
- •BSL-F, or fasting blood sugar, was 107 mg/dL (down from 120 mg/dL).
- 136 mg/dL was the postprandial blood sugar (PP) following the administration of the recommended medications.
- Weight: Dropped from 75 kg to 72 kg.

The patient was encouraged to stick to the naturopathy regimen while the dosage of the diabetic drug, Metformin, was decreased [51].

- **Results After a Few Months of Continued Therapy**

Following several months of ongoing care, the patient's condition improved:

Additional decrease in blood pressure to 125/85 mmHg.

- HBA1C: Dropped from 8.6% to 6.0%.
- Weight: Dropped from 75 kg to 67 kg.

This case study demonstrates the important role alternative medicines and naturopathy play in the treatment of Type 2 diabetes [51]. Dietary modifications, exercise, and home cures seem to have helped control blood pressure, lower weight, and regulate blood glucose levels [51]. Therefore, they help regulate diabetes and enhance general health by balancing the body's metabolism [51].

These data can be provided to various statistical and machine learning models that predict the blood glucose levels by incorporating the impact of alternative therapies along with lifestyle interventions for diabetes management. This can be a useful source for performing clinical trials and can also help identify potential drug targets.

CASE STUDY ON DATA-DRIVEN MODELING FOR DIABETES

Diabetes occurrence is predicted using a data-driven modeling technique, and patients are categorized based on risk variables. After the data is gathered, the best possible treatment regimens can be created, and healthcare researchers can make better decisions for people with diabetes. The introduction of data-driven models and their use in smarter and better diabetes management systems has been made possible by the growing availability of adequate patient history data. The success of models in diabetes research can be attributed to their ability to tackle complicated problems in a dynamic environment with information [52 - 54].

A case study of a data-driven method for parameter generation and verification in artificial pancreas control systems that provide insulin to people with type 1 diabetes (T1D) is presented in this work. The work presents a novel approach to control parameter adjustment by utilizing non-deterministic data-driven models for insulin-glucose regulation that are derived from patient data over a variety of time periods [52 - 54].

Participants: 50 anonymous T1D patients.

Sessions: 40 overnight sessions per patient.

Data Frequency: One-minute interval CGM readings.

Insulin Data: Detailed log of insulin delivered *via* a pump during each session.

Hypoglycaemia Events: Noted but not included in the dataset for modeling because of incomplete information on carbohydrate intake.

Exclusion of Early Data: To prevent confusion from the aftereffects of meals and exercise, the first 180 minutes of each nighttime session are eliminated. This guarantees that only the baseline dynamics of glucose and insulin are taken into account [52 - 54].

The study shows that a data-driven modeling approach helped predict the glucose-insulin dynamics. PID controllers were implemented to carry out the control algorithms that safely and reliably decide the insulin infusion rate based on glucose dynamics. The model can benefit clinical researchers to make quicker decisions, incorporating the whole day activity data along with variations in meals. It was concluded that these data-driven approaches can be used to make real-time predictions regarding the glucose dynamics.

CONCLUDING REMARKS

The healthcare sector has seen a significant transformation owing to *in silico* modeling and simulation techniques. Since *in silico* models provide a robust foundation for comprehending the intricate underlying mechanisms of insulin signaling pathways and, consequently, glucose regulation in diabetes, significant progress has been made in the management of the disease. Accurate and effective data can be produced using computational biotechnological technologies such as MATLAB, SimBiology, Simulink, Cell Designer, COPASI, and Multiphysics. The artificial pancreas and insulin infusion pumps are designed and developed with the use of these data. These models also account for the impact of drugs, lifestyle choices, diets, and alternative therapies on blood glucose levels. Therefore, data-driven model results can be used to recommend tailored treatment plans. Thus, personalized treatment strategies can be suggested based on data-driven model outcomes. *In silico* models not only contribute to providing in-depth knowledge of the physiology of diabetes but also provide valuable inputs to provide optimized treatment with advanced therapeutic innovations. With evolution, the integration of the *in silico* approach with *in vivo* and *in vitro* techniques contributes to providing faster and better research and clinical outcomes.

CONSENT FOR PUBLICATION

We hereby give consent for publication.

REFERENCES

[1]   MathWorks MATLAB (R2020b)

[2]   COPASI COPASI copasi.org

[3]   Funahashi A, Jouraku A, Matsuoka Y, Kitano H. Integration of CellDesigner and SABIO-RK. *In Silico* Biol. 2007;7(2 Suppl):S81–90. PMID: 17822394.

[4]   Buchwald P. COMSOL Multiphysics-based exploratory insulin secretion model for isolated pancreatic islets. Miami (FL): University of Miami; 2010.

[5]   Dalla Man C, Raimondo DM, Rizza RA, Cobelli C. GIM, simulation software of meal glucose-insulin model. J Diabetes Sci Technol 2007; 1(3): 323-30.
[http://dx.doi.org/10.1177/193229680700100303] [PMID: 19885087]

[6]   Mufti Azis M, Kristanto J, Sarto . Dynamic simulation of insulin-glucose interaction in type 1 diabetes with MATLAB Simulink® IOP Conference Series: Materials Science and Engineering. 2020.
[http://dx.doi.org/10.1088/1757-899X/778/1/012147]

[7]   Ferjouchia H, Iftahy FZ, Chadli A, *et al.* Application of optimal control strategies for physiological model of type 1 diabetes-t1d Commun Math Biol Neurosci 2020.
[http://dx.doi.org/10.28919/cmbn/4598]

[8]   Joshi DM. Dynamic *in silico* model of type 2 diabetes treated with metformin combined with exercise: A sobol sensitivity analysis 2022; 3 91-7.

[9]   Joshi DM, Patel J, Bhatt H. Dosage optimization of metformin and oleuropein along with exercise in diabetes management AIP Conference Proceedings. 2023.
[http://dx.doi.org/10.1063/5.0149280]

[10]   Ahmed J, Alvi BA, Khan ZA. Blood glucose-insulin regulation and management system using MATLAB/SIMULINK Proceedings - 4th IEEE International Conference on Emerging Technologies 2008, ICET 2008.
[http://dx.doi.org/10.1109/ICET.2008.4777519]

[11]   Isaac JS, Porkumaran K. Design of control technique for diabetes in critical care Proceeding of the IEEE International Conference on Green Computing, Communication and Electrical Engineering, ICGCCEE 2014.
[http://dx.doi.org/10.1109/ICGCCEE.2014.6922220]

[12]   Atanasijević-Kunc M, Drinovec J, Ručigaj S, Mrhar A. Modelling of the risk factors and chronic diseases that influence the development of serious health complications. Zdrav Vestn [Internet]. 2008 Aug   1   [cited   2026   Jan   16];77(8).   Available   from: https://vestnik.szd.si/index.php/ZdravVest/article/view/492

[13]   Vladimir B, Procofiev M, Komandresova T, *et al.* Modification of the minimal Bergman model of the 'insulin-glucose' system and its implementation in MatLab/Simulink Vide Tehnologija Resursi - Environment, Technology, Resources. 2021.
[http://dx.doi.org/10.17770/etr2021vol2.6659]

[14]   Pianosi F, Sarrazin F, Wagener T. A matlab toolbox for global sensitivity analysis. Environ Model Softw 2015; 70: 80-5.
[http://dx.doi.org/10.1016/j.envsoft.2015.04.009]

[15]   Wellock C, Chickarmane V, Sauro HM. The SBW–MATLAB interface. Bioinformatics 2005; 21(6): 823-4.
[http://dx.doi.org/10.1093/bioinformatics/bti110] [PMID: 15531613]

[16]   Park JS, Kim JR. Non-compartmental data analysis using SimBiology and MATLAB. Transl Clin Pharmacol 2019; 27(3): 89-91.
[http://dx.doi.org/10.12793/tcp.2019.27.3.89] [PMID: 32055588]

[17]   Ullah M, Schmidt H, Cho KH, *et al.* Deterministic modelling and stochastic simulation of biochemical pathways using MATLAB IEE Proc Syst Biol. 153
[http://dx.doi.org/10.1049/ip-syb:20050064]

[18]   Fundamentals of bioinformatics and computational biology: methods and exercises in MATLAB. Choice (Middletown) 2015; 52(9): 52-4752.
[http://dx.doi.org/10.5860/CHOICE.188432]

[19]   Bergmann FT, Hoops S, Klahn B, *et al.* COPASI and its applications in biotechnology. J Biotechnol 2017; 261: 215-20.
[http://dx.doi.org/10.1016/j.jbiotec.2017.06.1200] [PMID: 28655634]

[20]   Mendes P, Hoops S, Sahle S, Gauges R, Dada J, Kummer U. Computational modeling of biochemical networks using COPASI. Methods Mol Biol 2009; 500: 17-59.
[http://dx.doi.org/10.1007/978-1-59745-525-1_2] [PMID: 19399433]

[21]   Hoops S, Sahle S, Gauges R, *et al.* COPASI—a COmplex PAthway SImulator. Bioinformatics 2006; 22(24): 3067-74.
[http://dx.doi.org/10.1093/bioinformatics/btl485] [PMID: 17032683]

[22]   Bauerstätter P. Compartment modeling of overweight in toddler age: Modeling and simulating a diets effect with COPASI. SNE Simulation Notes Europe 2022; 32(4): 221-4.
[http://dx.doi.org/10.11128/sne.32.sn.10626]

[23]   Deepa Maheshvare M, Raha S, König M, Pal D. A pathway model of glucose-stimulated insulin secretion in the pancreatic β-cell. Front Endocrinol (Lausanne) 2023; 14: 1185656.
[http://dx.doi.org/10.3389/fendo.2023.1185656] [PMID: 37600713]

[24]   Kurlovics J, Zake DM, Zaharenko L, Berzins K, Klovins J, Stalidzans E. Metformin transport rates between plasma and red blood cells in humans. Clin Pharmacokinet 2022; 61(1): 133-42.
[http://dx.doi.org/10.1007/s40262-021-01058-2] [PMID: 34309806]

[25]   Joshi DM, Patel J, Bhatt H. *In silico* study to quantify the effect of exercise on surface GLUT4 translocation in diabetes management. Netw Model Anal Health Inform Bioinform 2021; 10(1): 1.
[http://dx.doi.org/10.1007/s13721-020-00274-3]

[26]   Joshi DM, Patel J, Bhatt H. Robust adaptation of PKC ζ-IRS1 insulin signaling pathways through integral feedback control. Biomed Phys Eng Express 2021; 7(5): 055013.
[http://dx.doi.org/10.1088/2057-1976/ac182e] [PMID: 34315137]

[27]   Funahashi A, Matsuoka Y, Jouraku A, Morohashi M, Kikuchi N, Kitano H. CellDesigner 3.5: A versatile modeling tool for biochemical networks. Proc IEEE 2008; 96(8): 1254-65.
[http://dx.doi.org/10.1109/JPROC.2008.925458]

[28]   Matsuoka Y, Funahashi A, Ghosh S, Kitano H. Modeling and simulation using CellDesigner. Methods Mol Biol 2014; 1164: 121-45.
[http://dx.doi.org/10.1007/978-1-4939-0805-9_11] [PMID: 24927840]

[29]   Kwei E, Sanft K, Petzold L, *et al. Systems analysis of the insulin signaling pathway.* IFAC 2008.
[http://dx.doi.org/10.3182/20080706-5-KR-1001.02686]

[30]   Sedaghat AR, Sherman A, Quon MJ. A mathematical model of metabolic insulin signaling pathways. Am J Physiol Endocrinol Metab 2002; 283(5): E1084-101.
[http://dx.doi.org/10.1152/ajpendo.00571.2001] [PMID: 12376338]

[31]   Pareek A, Mathur T, Runkana V, *et al.* Mathematical modeling of glucose responsive hydrogels Tech Pap Present by COMSOL 2015; pp. 4-6.

[32]   Marra V. Bringing glucose monitoring to new levels through integrated sensor design, Med Design Briefs 2018.

[33]   Paavola CD, Allen DP, Shekhawat D, *et al.* ADME Properties of Insulins The ADME Encyclopedia. 2022.
[http://dx.doi.org/10.1007/978-3-030-84860-6_121]

[34]   Chen W, Lu J, Plum-Mörschel L, *et al.* Pharmacokinetic and pharmacodynamic bioequivalence of Gan & Lee insulin analogues aspart (rapilin®), lispro (prandilin®) and glargine (basalin®) with EU - und US□SOURCED reference insulins. Diabetes Obes Metab 2023; 25(12): 3817-25.
[http://dx.doi.org/10.1111/dom.15281] [PMID: 37735841]

[35]   Muise ES, Guan HP, Liu J, *et al.* Pharmacological AMPK activation induces transcriptional responses

congruent to exercise in skeletal and cardiac muscle, adipose tissues and liver. PLoS One 2019; 14(2): e0211568.
[http://dx.doi.org/10.1371/journal.pone.0211568] [PMID: 30811418]

[36]   Daskalaki A. *Handbook of research on systems biology applications in medicine.* 2008.
[http://dx.doi.org/10.4018/978-1-60566-076-9]

[37]   de Oliveira LEC, da Silva LA, Wouk J, *et al.* Role of AMPK and its possible interactions in metformin therapy and physical exercise-Research perspectives. J Appl Pharm Sci 2017; 7: 196-9.

[38]   Summer T. *Sensitivity Analysis in Systems Biology Modelling and its Application to a Multi-Scale Model of Blood Glucose Homeostasis* http://eprints.ucl.ac.uk/19896/1/19896.pdf2010.

[39]   Joshi T, Singh AK, Haratipour P, *et al.* Targeting AMPK signaling pathway by natural products for treatment of diabetes mellitus and its complications. J Cell Physiol 2019; 234(10): 17212-31.
[http://dx.doi.org/10.1002/jcp.28528] [PMID: 30916407]

[40]   Steinberg GR, Carling D. AMP-activated protein kinase: the current landscape for drug development. Nat Rev Drug Discov 2019; 18(7): 527-51.
[http://dx.doi.org/10.1038/s41573-019-0019-2] [PMID: 30867601]

[41]   Stepensky D, Friedman M, Raz I, Hoffman A. Pharmacokinetic-pharmacodynamic analysis of the glucose-lowering effect of metformin in diabetic rats reveals first-pass pharmacodynamic effect. Drug Metab Dispos 2002; 30(8): 861-8.
[http://dx.doi.org/10.1124/dmd.30.8.861] [PMID: 12124302]

[42]   Scheen AJ. Clinical pharmacokinetics of metformin. Clin Pharmacokinet 1996; 30(5): 359-71.
[http://dx.doi.org/10.2165/00003088-199630050-00003] [PMID: 8743335]

[43]   Pearson ER. Personalized medicine in diabetes: the role of 'omics' and biomarkers. Diabet Med 2016; 33(6): 712-7.
[http://dx.doi.org/10.1111/dme.13075] [PMID: 26802434]

[44]   Semiz S, Dujic T, Causevic A. Pharmacogenetics and personalized treatment of type 2 diabetes. Biochem Med (Zagreb) 2013; 23(2): 154-71.
[http://dx.doi.org/10.11613/BM.2013.020] [PMID: 23894862]

[45]   Hu C. Pharmacogenomics in type 2 diabetes management: towards personalized medicine. J Transl Med 2012; 10(S2): A19.
[http://dx.doi.org/10.1186/1479-5876-10-S2-A19]

[46]   El Youssef J, Castle J, Ward WK. A review of closed-loop algorithms for glycemic control in the treatment of type 1 diabetes. Algorithms 2009; 2(1): 518-32.
[http://dx.doi.org/10.3390/a2010518]

[47]   Heinemann L. Variability of insulin absorption and insulin action. Diabetes Technol Ther 2002; 4(5): 673-82.
[http://dx.doi.org/10.1089/152091502320798312] [PMID: 12450450]

[48]   Arnolds S, Kuglin B, Kapitza C, Heise T. How pharmacokinetic and pharmacodynamic principles pave the way for optimal basal insulin therapy in type 2 diabetes. Int J Clin Pract 2010; 64(10): 1415-24.
[http://dx.doi.org/10.1111/j.1742-1241.2010.02470.x] [PMID: 20618882]

[49]   Lin S, Chien YW. Pharmacokinetic-pharmacodynamic modelling of insulin: Comparison of indirect pharmacodynamic response with effect-compartment link models. J Pharm Pharmacol 2002; 54(6): 791-800.
[http://dx.doi.org/10.1211/0022357021779131] [PMID: 12078995]

[50]   Freil KS, Fritzen LO, Boiroux D, Aradottir TB, Jørgensen JB. Identification of PK-PD Insulin Models using Experimental GIR Data. IFAC-PapersOnLine 2024; 58(24): 484-9.
[http://dx.doi.org/10.1016/j.ifacol.2024.11.085]

[51]   Faggionato E, Schiavon M, Dalla Man C. Modeling between-subject variability in subcutaneous absorption of a fast-acting insulin analogue by a nonlinear mixed effects approach. Metabolites 2021; 11(4): 235.
[http://dx.doi.org/10.3390/metabo11040235] [PMID: 33921274]

[52]   Zhang Y, Holt TA, Khovanova N. A data driven nonlinear stochastic model for blood glucose dynamics. Comput Methods Programs Biomed 2016; 125: 18-25.
[http://dx.doi.org/10.1016/j.cmpb.2015.10.021] [PMID: 26707373]

[53]   Woldaregay AZ, Årsand E, Walderhaug S, *et al.* Data-driven modeling and prediction of blood glucose dynamics: Machine learning applications in type 1 diabetes. Artif Intell Med 2019; 98: 109-34.
[http://dx.doi.org/10.1016/j.artmed.2019.07.007] [PMID: 31383477]

[54]   Dinh A, Miertschin S, Young A, Mohanty SD. A data-driven approach to predicting diabetes and cardiovascular disease with machine learning. BMC Med Inform Decis Mak 2019; 19(1): 211.
[http://dx.doi.org/10.1186/s12911-019-0918-5] [PMID: 31694707]

CHAPTER 5

Applications of *In Silico* Modeling in Diabetes Therapy

Abstract: With the increasing prevalence of type 1 and type 2 diabetes, management, particularly for those receiving insulin therapy, becomes a global health concern. Since the advancement of *in silico* models, diabetes treatment has greatly improved. Computer simulations forecast the insulin dosages needed for bolus and basal infusion based on real-time glucose dynamics. By replicating glucose-insulin dynamics and taking into account factors like age, activity, food intake, insulin resistance, and more, these models—like the UVA/PADOVA simulator—have completely changed the way people with diabetes are treated. These algorithms not only forecast insulin dosages but also help with medication customization, thereby improving patient outcomes. When factors like stress and physical activity are taken into account, *in silico* models offer vital information on the ideal basal and bolus insulin dosages. Additionally, even in the absence of exact insulin-to-carbohydrate ratios, reinforcement learning models have demonstrated potential in predicting bolus insulin doses, increasing the accuracy of insulin delivery. Despite improvements, data validation, device integration, and the requirement for individualized care continue to pose challenges to these models' ability to accurately forecast insulin dosages. Several *in silico* modeling techniques, their uses, and the significance of tailored care in maximizing diabetes management are covered in this research.

Keywords: Diabetes, *In silico*, Insulin dose, Insulin therapy, Personalized treatment, Simulation.

INTRODUCTION

Type 1 and Type 2 diabetes are important global health threats affecting millions of people across the world. This is an issue that is seeing increasing numbers every day, and therefore, finding effective strategies to manage this will always be necessary. One of the biggest areas of concern for people suffering from type 1 and many type 2 diabetes patients is how to maintain blood glucose levels with insulin dosage. Insulin therapy is a primary treatment method for both forms of diabetes, but the timing, dose, and how it is given are extremely critical. The mismanaged insulin dosage is a significant weakness of the older systems that relied on fixed protocols or basic mechanistic models, as they do not consider the level of sophistication and complexity of the glucose-insulin relationship in the

Darshna M. Joshi, Hardik Bhatt & Himanshu K. Patel

human body. The past few years have seen a paradigm shift in diabetes treatment with the emergence of *in silico* models, which are computer-based biological systems. These models are now able to simulate the human body in real time, ensuring individual attention is needed for effective bolus and basal insulin infusions. These models are able to incorporate various other determinants like a person's age, level of activity, food consumption, insulin tolerance, and more, which greatly aids in the more complex task of insulin control.

To put models like the UVA/PADOVA simulator in simpler terms, they have shifted treatment strategies for these chronic conditions from a standard treatment approach to a more individualized treatment approach. *In silico* methods not only estimate insulin requirements but also aid in forecasting other medication schedules, which enhances the outcome and quality of life for patients. These models capture daily changes, including stress, physical activity, and meal intake, which allows for on-the-spot insulin administration decisions. Furthermore, novel methods, like those using reinforcement learning, have also emerged that are highly accurate in anticipating bolus delivery of insulin based on predetermined factors, with no precise carbohydrate-to-insulin ratio required.

In spite of these advancements, progress has been hampered by several issues. The accuracy of data validation, along with the integration of various data sources and the customization of treatment, is an ongoing challenge. In addition, patient privacy and the clinical relevance of these models in practice pose significant challenges to their broader utilization. This chapter will cover *in silico* modeling methods in diabetes care, considering their challenges, benefits, and the new possibilities that have emerged with them. The chapter aims to summarize how insulin therapy can be optimized, and consequently, how the life of a diabetic patient can greatly improve through *in silico* modeling. The significance of customizing treatment protocols for individual patients, as well as the need to improve these models for general clinical application, will be discussed.

IN SILICO MODELS' BASAL INSULIN INFUSION RATES AND BOLUS DOSES

Diabetes management is a global matter of worry these days. It is predicted by the International Diabetes Federation and the World Health Organization that if proper attention is not given, the world will surely enter into a diabetes epidemic soon. Computational techniques have revolutionized the world today, with the ability to simulate complex biological behaviors and predict outcomes in no time. *In silico* models, such as computational and mathematical models, are built to simulate the glucose-insulin dynamics of the body. These models, therefore, enhance the lives of diabetic patients on insulin therapy by making accurate predictions regarding the basal and bolus doses of insulin infusion on the basis of glucose levels in the body.

Basal insulin is required to maintain the glucose levels in the body throughout the day and night. This dose covers the metabolic needs of the body when no diet is followed. Usually, long-acting insulin injections are used to deliver insulin. However, bolus insulin is required when there is a sudden rise in glucose levels due to meals. Rapid-acting insulin injections are preferred in such cases. The optimum dose of basal or bolus insulin is decided by advanced *in silico* models that take into account various factors of the body, such as age, weight, digestive speed, exercise, insulin resistance, and more. There are various types of *in silico* models available, like empirical models, mechanistic models, physiological models, and minimal models. In this section, we will discuss three *in silico* models used to deliver basal insulin infusion and bolus doses.

Enrique *et al.* [1] used the recently developed type 1 diabetes simulator called UVA/PADOVA [2, 3], which provides a realistic testing scenario to determine the basal insulin infusion and bolus dose based on glucose-insulin dynamics of individuals. The simulator has generated more than 100 *in silico* diabetes patients' simulations and predicted the doses accurately.

This led to the acceptance of the simulator by the Food and Drug Administration (FDA). The sample model is shown in Fig.(**1**). Advanced diabetes technologies like artificial pancreas systems, glucose sensors, and new insulin molecules can be tested with the simulator. Enrique *et al.* generated a virtual patient, and new rules to find the insulin-to-Carbohydrate Ratio (CR) and Correction Factors (CF) have been introduced.

The simulation is implemented in MATLAB, where the user can select basic details like meal timing, carbohydrate amounts, age, and number of patients. One can even select the hardware, such as glucose sensors and insulin infusion pumps. Furthermore, the route of insulin infusion is selected, and the simulation is allowed to run, where glucose control dynamics are available in terms of graphs and values. The impact of variations during meals or exercise is taken into account, and the simulator provides the basal and bolus doses of insulin required to maintain glucose levels under regulation. The simulation is run for hours overnight to determine the doses. The results require further study, but are instructive for clinical trials, facilitating faster and better decision-making for patients with type 1 diabetes.

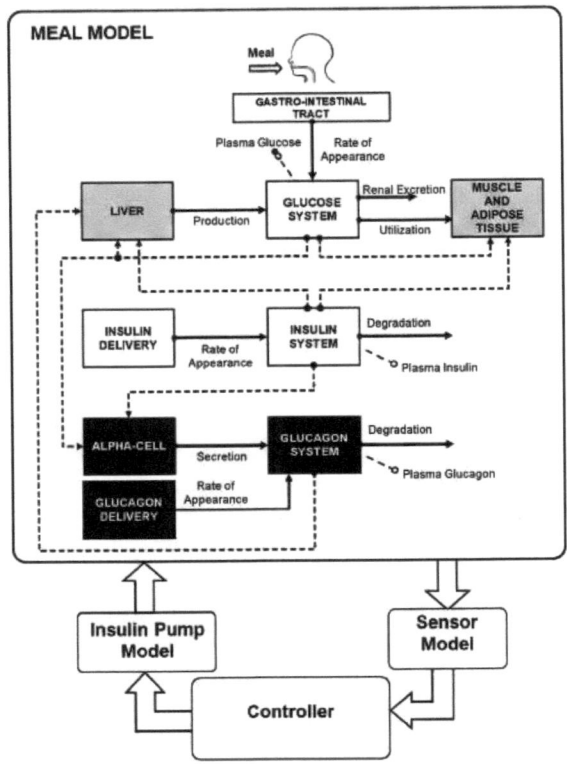

Fig. (1). UVA/PADOVA type 1 diabetes simulator [3].

Moving further, Michele *et al.* [4] explored an interesting *in silico* model based on the optimization of basal insulin infusion when exercise is performed. It is discussed that when physical activity is done, glucose dynamics are considered by *in silico* models, and artificial pancreas systems are thus instructed to release basal insulin according to control algorithms in closed-loop control. They have presented a modified version of the UVA/PADOVA Type 1 diabetes simulator, as shown in Fig.(**2**), by incorporating the effect of exercise.

Insulin sensitivity is tested under both resting and exercise conditions, and it has been found that exercise enhances insulin sensitivity. Virtual patients were simulated with varying basal insulin rates, and results were observed. The model predicted a reduction in basal insulin of almost 50% if physical activity is performed. The insulin reduction pattern of the patient should be taken as an important input to the control algorithm of an artificial pancreas when deciding the insulin infusion rate.

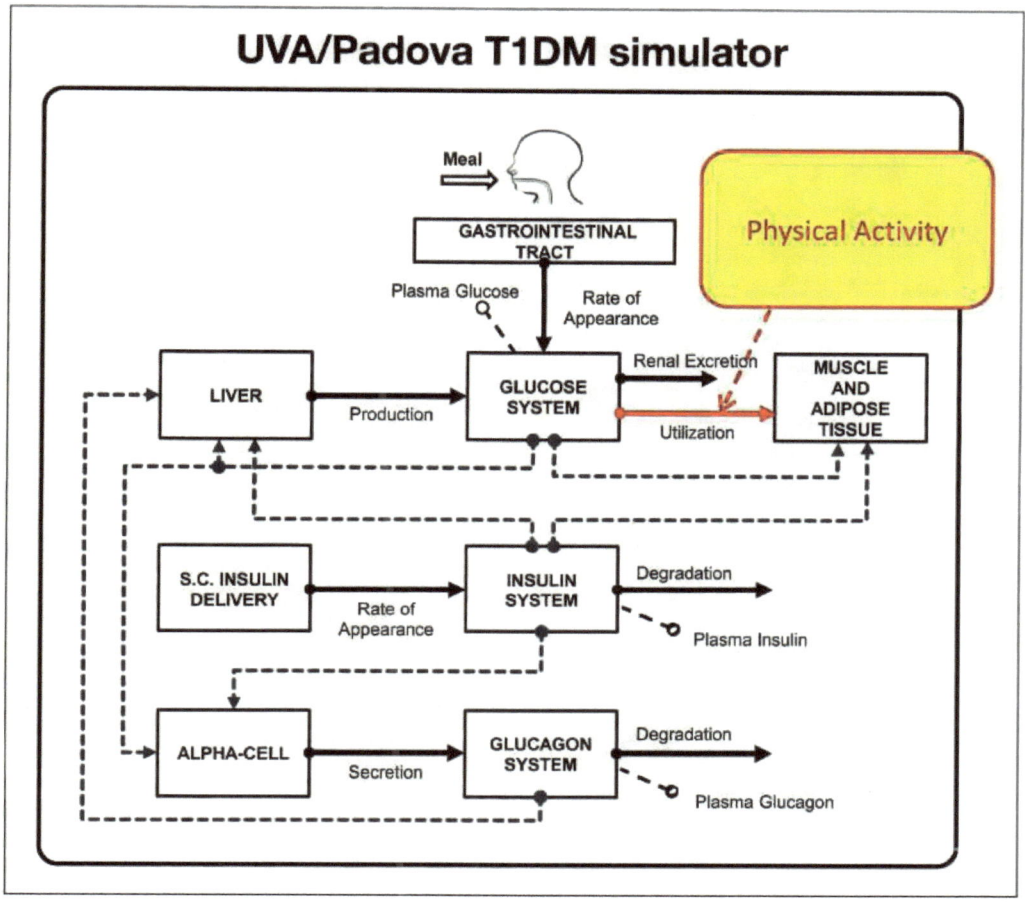

Fig. (2). New Version of UVA/PADOVA type 1 diabetes simulator [4].

The purpose of this model is to suggest the optimum basal insulin dose when clinical trials for type 1 diabetes are performed that include physical exercise. The results satisfactorily demonstrate the importance of physical exercise in the reduction of the insulin dose required to maintain glucose levels in the body. A safe and effective basal insulin dose strategy is suggested for diabetes management.

Furthermore, the basal insulin infusion and bolus doses are determined based on factors like insulin-to-carbohydrate ratio, carbohydrate intake, and other correction factors. If there are any errors in identifying these variables, the chances are that the burden of overdosing on insulin or the risk of lesser insulin against the required dose increases. Sayyar *et al.* [5] presented a Q-learning-based technique that uses reinforcement learning and can predict the optimum bolus dose without being dependent on the factors mentioned above. The pictorial representation of the model developed is shown in Fig.(**3**).

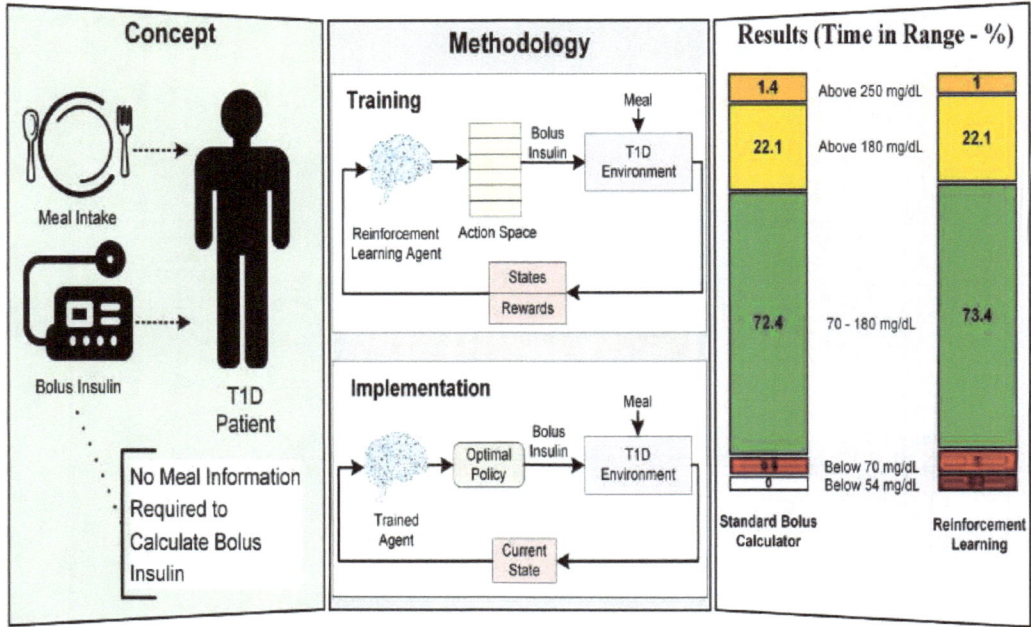

Fig. (3). Reinforcement learning model for boulus insulin dose prediction [5].

In silico trials were carried out using a virtual cohort of 68 patients [5]. The results were validated by comparing them to standard bolus calculators available. As expected, when errors in calculating the ratios or factors were present, the reinforcement model predicted accurate results in comparison to standard calculators. Also, in normal conditions, the results were similar to standard bolus calculators [5]. It is thus recommended that this algorithm be incorporated into an artificial pancreas system to automate insulin delivery in an optimal way.

Although such advancements in *in silico* modeling have helped significantly in diabetes management, model validation and the applicability of the results to a variety of patients are significant challenges. The collection of data from various devices like sensors, glucose monitors, physical activity, medications, and others to better predict the insulin dose remains a tough job. Additionally, the control algorithms are improving day by day, which remains another challenge to cope with glucose dynamics under various conditions and individual characteristics. It is expected that a collective model incorporating various real factors, such as the impact of stress, yoga, and meditation, will be included in the model to accurately balance the insulin dose required for glucose regulation.

IMPACT OF MINIMAL INSULIN DOSES ON BLOOD GLUCOSE LEVELS

Optimal glucose control is the utmost requirement of type 1 or type 2 diabetic patients. When insulin is necessary for the patient, it becomes a tedious task to administer insulin injections daily as per the recommended units based on the variations in blood glucose levels. Hence, the dose of insulin is an important factor to be considered for research and the application of diabetes management. The minimum quantity of insulin needed to successfully control blood glucose levels in order to reduce the risk of hyperglycaemia or hypoglycaemia and prevent consequences is referred to as the minimal insulin dose [6 - 12].

Glucose homeostasis in the body is maintained by a sufficient amount of insulin available and the response of other physiological processes. For each individual, the minimal dose of insulin varies based on insulin sensitivity, physical exercise, medications, food habits, and the metabolism of the body. As explained in the previous section, basal and bolus doses of insulin refer to the amount of insulin required in a fasting and meal-taking state, respectively, in patients. Hence, an insulin dose is required in a lesser amount when a person has lower insulin resistance, while a higher dose is needed when organs are insulin-insensitive for glucose control. The type of diet consumed decides the bolus dose of insulin. Physical exercise of different intensity also has an impact on the insulin dose [13 - 22].

Additionally, the pharmacokinetics of insulin plays a crucial role in preventing the fluctuations in blood glucose. If the dose is less than glucose production, one may suffer from hyperglycaemia (high blood glucose levels), which increases diabetic complications. Similarly, too much insulin, even if minimal, leads to hypoglycemia (low blood glucose). Hence, an optimal insulin level is significant in the maintenance of glucose levels. There are two concentrations of regular human insulin available: 100 units per millilitre (U-100) and 500 units per millilitre (U-500). Individualized dosages should be determined by the patient's metabolic requirements, blood glucose readings, and glycemic objectives. The typical range for daily insulin needs is 0.5 to 1 unit/kg [23 - 26].

Additionally, when the minimal dose is used, one may face frequent fluctuations in blood glucose levels if food intake is not balanced. For type 1 diabetes patients, insulin is not produced in the body itself; hence, a sufficient dose is required. In the case of type 2 diabetes, insulin is produced to some extent in the body, and hence, the minimal dose will be different in such cases. If patients start exercising, the insulin requirement by the body will be reduced, and the minimal dose will change accordingly. Hence, a minimal insulin dose has a critical impact on the regulation of blood glucose levels [26 - 28].

Sujay *et al.* [29] and Leslie *et al.* [30] demonstrated the role of insulin in the management of type 2 diabetes mellitus. They have shown various insulin types available and the pharmacokinetics of the insulin for various categories of patients involved. The pharmacological action of insulin is discussed, and recommendations for insulin based on an individual's characteristics are suggested. It is shown that glucose levels are recorded in the initial few weeks in response to insulin dose variations, and finally, a minimal dose of insulin is decided based on clinical experiences. The commonly used terms in deciding insulin dose are shown in Table **1**.

Table 1. Commonly used terms in insulin therapy.

Term	Definition	Calculation
Augmentation	Use of either basal or bolus insulin to help improve glucose control in patients with partial beta-cell failure.	0.3 unit per kg
Replacement	Use of basal and bolus insulin to control blood glucose when endogenous insulin production is minimal or absent.	0.6 to 1.0 unit per kg
Carbohydrate ratio	The number of units of insulin needed to cover a certain number of grams of carbohydrates ingested.	500 divided by total daily insulin (usually about 1 unit per 10g)
Correction (sensitivity)	How much 1 unit of insulin is expected to decrease the patient's blood glucose level when the blood glucose level is above predefined targets. Short-acting insulin may be added to the bolus dose or given separately between meals.	1,500 divided by total daily insulin (usually about 1 unit per 25g)

The management of insulin in type 2 diabetes has been studied by Amanda *et al.* [27]. A detailed explanation of the process used to determine insulin therapy is provided. The American Diabetes Association and the European Association for the Study of Diabetes (EASD) have made an intriguing proposal regarding insulin therapy. The flowchart in Fig. (**4**) gives information about the selection of insulin dosage that aids in the management of diabetes based on a number of variables, including age, weight, and eating habits. Insulin therapy decisions are based on continuous glucose monitoring devices. Bolus insulin dosage and insulin-to-carbohydrate ratios are computed. In order to minimize blood glucose variations and administer an adequate quantity of insulin in a precise manner, regulated insulin infusion pumps are utilized. Long-term issues can be avoided by making decisions based on individual factors, which improves overall health results.

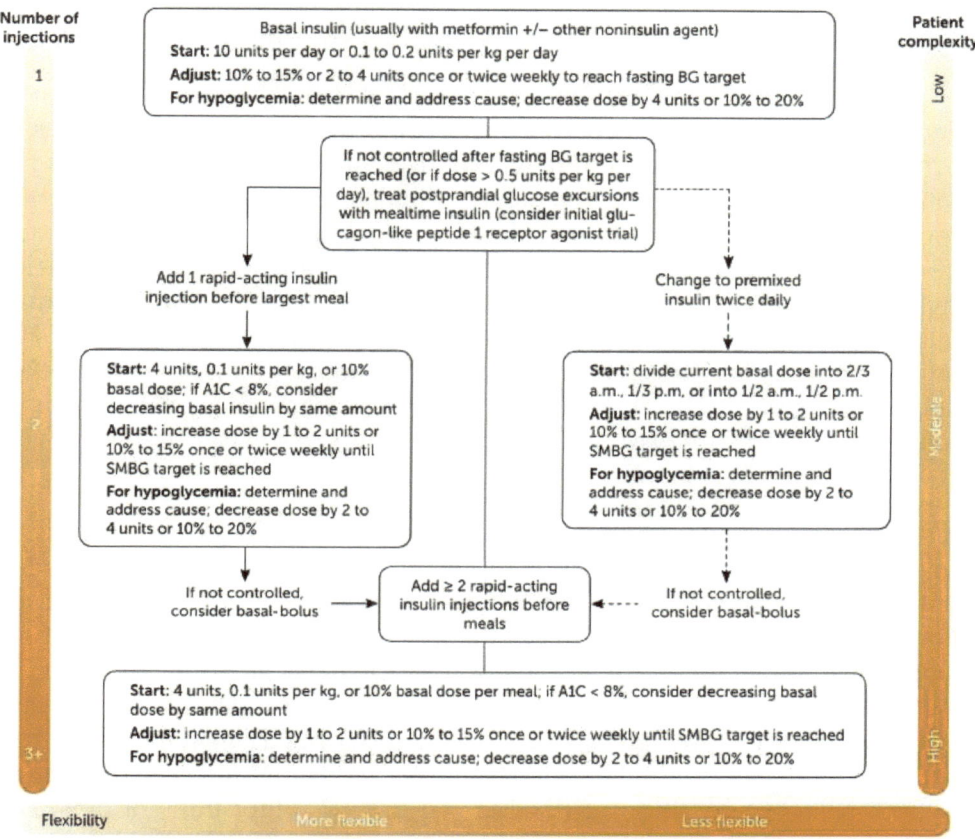

Fig. (4). Insulin dose therapy [27].

PERSONALIZED DIABETES MANAGEMENT: *IN SILICO* MODELING

With the global diabetes epidemic, technological advancements are desperately needed. Several physiological traits must be taken into account when managing the onset of diabetes. Approaches to glucose regulation treatment must be tailored to each patient's situation. Therefore, customized treatment is the best way to properly regulate blood glucose levels. Factors such as genetics, physical activity, diet, smoking, yoga, meditation, stress, and others are considered when designing a personalized therapy plan. This makes it possible to produce diabetic medications with a more effective target-based approach. Computational models require precise data or a sizable dataset in order to provide individualized treatment. The intricate underlying mechanism of the insulin signaling pathway should be taken into account by the model. The *in silico* model's capacity to deliver individualized care enhances with the level of pathway construction. Furthermore, people with diabetes may also have additional conditions that should be taken into account while evaluating the model to determine the objectives [31 - 37].

Traditionally, trial-and-error techniques were employed together with drugs such as metformin, where the effects of diet, exercise, and lifestyle choices could only be evaluated in clinical trials. By creating and building diabetes models that incorporate minute details of many disease characteristics, along with external inputs like lifestyle and diet, *in silico* models have increased the complexity of research. Consequently, it may be possible to create individualized treatment plans that use glucose levels to determine the appropriate insulin dosage. Based on patient-specific data, these models are able to forecast long-term results based on glucose dynamics. The main benefit is that, because it is a computational method, results from *in silico* models can be employed instead of expensive and time-consuming *in vitro* and *in vivo* research [33, 38, 39].

Lehel *et al.* [40] showed a personalized treatment strategy based on reinforcement learning algorithms. In order to overcome the drawbacks of conventional techniques that are not flexible, this study investigates the possibility of using Reinforcement Learning (RL) to develop customized blood glucose management programs. A mathematical model customized for patients with type 1 diabetes was created as part of the study, and it was verified using data from ten patients and seventeen key parameters. To simulate real-world circumstances, the model included elements like random carbohydrate consumption and noise from Continuous Glucose Monitoring (CGM). To use RL algorithms, a closed-loop system was developed, employing a Policy Optimization (PPO) methodology. An average Time in Range (TIR) of 73% was found in the data, indicating better blood glucose control. With significant implications for tailored care, the study emphasizes the promise of RL-based personalized insulin administration as a viable way to improve diabetes management.

Fatemah *et al.* [41] carried out a study that uses digital twins and Personal Health Knowledge Graphs (PHKGs) to present a novel method for managing diabetes. The foundation of this approach is a patient-centered, real-time digital twin structure that complies with HL7 standards to guarantee accurate and smooth information flow while integrating data from several sources. As more information becomes available, PHKGs offer a scalable and adaptable framework for incorporating new patient data, thereby improving the accuracy of care. Patient care can be updated and improved continuously thanks to this dynamic system. Several diabetes care tasks, including glucose level prediction, insulin dosage optimization, tailored lifestyle recommendations, and health data visualization, were used to illustrate the framework's adaptability. The digital twin framework is shown in Fig.(**5**).

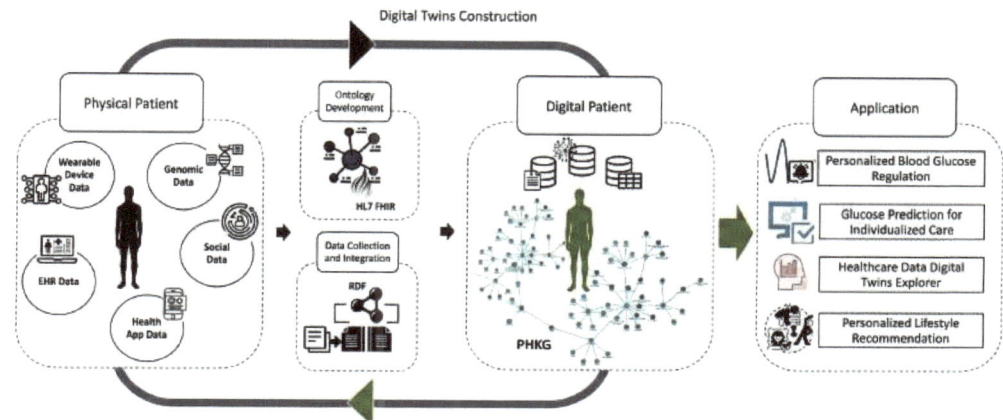

Fig. (5). Digital twin model [41].

Jinyu *et al.* [42] investigated the short-term and long-term effects of Physical Activity (PA) on insulin-independent glucose fluctuation and insulin sensitivity. This research proposes a data-driven model for glucose dynamics that takes PA into account. Both a linear regression of PA and a bilinear regression of insulin and PA are included in the suggested nonlinear model with physical activity (NLPA). Data from a physiological PA-glucose model by Dalla Man *et al.*, combined with the UVA/PADOVA Simulator, was used to assess the model's performance. The findings demonstrated that the NLPA and a linear model with PA (LPA) performed better than a model without PA (LOPA), with 45–180% higher goodness of fit for short-term glucose predictions (30 minutes ahead). When no past measures were used, NLPA showed an 87% better fit than LPA in terms of the long-term effects of PA on insulin sensitivity. Furthermore, NLPA outperformed LPA and LOPA by 25–37% in predicting post-exercise hypoglycaemia. According to this study, taking into consideration the effects of PA, especially its long-term impacts on insulin sensitivity, can increase the accuracy of glucose predictions and aid in better anticipating post-exercise hypoglycemia. Additional human trials will be necessary to validate these findings.

Jinyu *et al.* [43] showed that to minimize hypoglycemia episodes and attain ideal glycemic control, individuals with Type 1 Diabetes (T1D) need individualized nutrition and exercise management. For T1D patients, this study developed a model-based recommender system that provides customized exercise and food regimens. By minimizing a risk function over a future time horizon, the system forecasts blood glucose levels using a patient-specific model of glucose dynamics and then suggests tailored actions, including meal/snack amounts or target heart rates during exercise. Based on a modified UVA/PADOVA simulator with an additional exercise-glucose subsystem, simulations involving 30 virtual individuals revealed that the Recommender performed better than the Starter and Skilled schemes, two self-management strategies. The Recommender performed similarly to the Skilled scheme, lowering the Mean Low Blood Glucose Index by 84% and the Blood Glucose Risk Index by 49% ($P < 0.05$). It also reduced the frequency of hypoglycaemia episodes during and after exercise, suggesting that it may help manage type 1 diabetes.

Kirill *et al.* [44] showed that one of the main goals of research on diabetes mellitus treatment is to develop a closed-loop system for blood glucose control. The control method presented in this paper is intended to keep blood glucose levels within a physiological range. The controller has an optimal bolus calculation and proportional regulation for automatic modification of the basal insulin infusion rate. It incorporates meal data, ongoing blood glucose monitoring, and individualized patient data, including insulin sensitivity and basal insulin infusion rate. The UVA/Padova type 1 diabetes simulator, which simulates both glucose metabolism and insulin pump dynamics, was used to test the suggested method *in silico*. The algorithm's potential for use in a closed-loop blood glucose control system was suggested by the encouraging results of simulations of 24-hour closed-loop regulation that included four meals per day for nine adults and ten adolescents.

Long-term diabetes progression can be predicted and simulated utilizing *in silico* models that take individual features into consideration. With simulators, virtual patients can be created and given a range of traits and lifestyle choices. As a result, insulin and other medication dosages can be optimized. It is feasible to predict the effects of varying insulin dosages on blood glucose levels and eliminate costly and time-consuming trial-and-error methods. The models must accurately capture the intricacy of human physiology, which is a difficult undertaking. To date, no simulation model has been able to account for all biological parameters. Additionally, a significant amount of patient data must be handled carefully, and privacy must be preserved. Even when simulation findings are good, clinical validation of the model and its outcome is necessary for people to receive dependable and efficient treatment. These days, AI and ML models are developing quickly to produce accurate forecasts and simulations for glucose regulation in the treatment of diabetes. Thus, personalized diabetes management is a worthwhile approach that can be achieved through *in silico* modeling.

CONCLUDING REMARKS

With its ability to anticipate and customize insulin administration, *in silico* modeling has become a game-changing tool in the treatment of diabetes. Effective methods for simulating glucose-insulin dynamics and figuring out the best basal and bolus insulin dosages under varied physiological conditions include models such as the UVA/PADOVA simulator and reinforcement learning-based approaches. In addition to increasing insulin administration accuracy, these models make it easier to incorporate lifestyle aspects like exercise and dietary habits into diabetes treatment plans. However, model validation, integrating data from multiple sources, and protecting patient privacy are still major obstacles. Future studies should concentrate on enhancing model robustness by including more individual characteristics that affect glucose control, such as stress, sleep, and mental health.

The ultimate objective is to shift toward a more individualized strategy for managing diabetes by utilizing *in silico* models' skills to optimize insulin dosages and reduce the likelihood of hypoglycemia or hyperglycemia. Even if these models have a lot of potential, their clinical use needs to be thoroughly verified through extensive trials to guarantee their reliability and effectiveness in actual diabetic treatment.

CONSENT FOR PUBLICATION

We hereby give consent for publication.

REFERENCES

[1]   Campos-Náñez E, Layne JE, Zisser HC. *In silico* modeling of minimal effective insulin doses using the UVA/PADOVA type 1 diabetes simulator. J Diabetes Sci Technol. 2018; 12.
[http://dx.doi.org/10.1177/1932296817735341]

[2]   Visentin R, Campos-Náñez E, Schiavon M, *et al.* The UVA/Padova type 1 diabetes simulator goes from single meal to single day. J Diabetes Sci Technol 2018; 12(2): 273-81.
[http://dx.doi.org/10.1177/1932296818757747] [PMID: 29451021]

[3]   Man CD, Micheletto F, Lv D, Breton M, Kovatchev B, Cobelli C. The UVA/PADOVA type 1 diabetes simulator: New features. J Diabetes Sci Technol 2014; 8(1): 26-34.
[http://dx.doi.org/10.1177/1932296813514502] [PMID: 24876534]

[4]   Schiavon M, Man CD, Kudva YC, Basu A, Cobelli C. *In silico* optimization of basal insulin infusion rate during exercise: implication for artificial pancreas. J Diabetes Sci Technol 2013; 7(6): 1461-9.
[http://dx.doi.org/10.1177/193229681300700606] [PMID: 24351172]

[5]   Ahmad S, Beneyto A, Contreras I, Vehi J. Bolus Insulin calculation without meal information. A reinforcement learning approach. Artif Intell Med 2022; 134: 102436.

[http://dx.doi.org/10.1016/j.artmed.2022.102436] [PMID: 36462903]

[6]   Garige M, Ghosh S, Roelofs B, Rao VA, Sourbier C. Protocol to assess the biological activity of insulin glargine, insulin lispro, and insulin aspart *in vitro*. Methods Protoc 2023; 6(2): 33.
[http://dx.doi.org/10.3390/mps6020033] [PMID: 37104015]

[7]   Marks J. Insulin analogues. Postgrad Med 2002; 112(5) (Suppl Designer): 8-12.
[http://dx.doi.org/10.3810/pgm.1997.02.157] [PMID: 19667599]

[8]   Insulin-aspart/insulin-glargine/insulin-lispro Reactions Weekly 18042020;
[http://dx.doi.org/10.1007/s40278-020-78588-9]

[9]   Morettini M, Palumbo MC, Göbl C, *et al.* Mathematical model of insulin kinetics accounting for the amino acids effect during a mixed meal tolerance test. Front Endocrinol (Lausanne) 2022; 13: 966305.
[http://dx.doi.org/10.3389/fendo.2022.966305] [PMID: 36187117]

[10] Siebenhofer A, Plank J, Berghold A, *et al.* Short acting insulin analogues *versus* regular human insulin in patients with diabetes mellitus. Cochrane Libr 2006; (2): CD003287.
[http://dx.doi.org/10.1002/14651858.CD003287.pub4] [PMID: 16625575]

[11] Fullerton B, Siebenhofer A, Jeitler K, *et al.* Short-acting insulin analogues *versus* regular human insulin for adult, non-pregnant persons with type 2 diabetes mellitus. Cochrane Database of Systematic Reviews 2018.
[http://dx.doi.org/10.1002/14651858.CD013228]

[12] Malek R, Davis SN. Novel methods of insulin replacement: The artificial pancreas and encapsulated islets. Rev Recent Clin Trials 2016; 11(2): 106-23.
[http://dx.doi.org/10.2174/1574887111666151207112100] [PMID: 26638972]

[13] Heinemann L. Variability of insulin absorption and insulin action. Diabetes Technol Ther 2002; 4(5): 673-82.
[http://dx.doi.org/10.1089/152091502320798312] [PMID: 12450450]

[14] Vardi M, Jacobson E, Nini A, Bitterman H. Intermediate acting versus long acting insulin for type 1 diabetes mellitus. Cochrane Libr 2008; 2008(3): CD006297.
[http://dx.doi.org/10.1002/14651858.CD006297.pub2] [PMID: 18646147]

[15] Faggionato E, Schiavon M, Dalla Man C. Modeling between-subject variability in subcutaneous absorption of a fast-acting insulin analogue by a nonlinear mixed effects approach. Metabolites 2021; 11(4): 235.
[http://dx.doi.org/10.3390/metabo11040235] [PMID: 33921274]

[16] Paavola CD, Allen DP, Shekhawat D, *et al.* ADME properties of insulins. The ADME Encyclopedia. 2022.
[http://dx.doi.org/10.1007/978-3-030-84860-6_121]

[17] Mufti Azis M, Kristanto J, Sarto . Dynamic simulation of insulin-glucose interaction in type 1 diabetes with MATLAB Simulink® IOP Conference Series: Materials Science and Engineering.
[http://dx.doi.org/10.1088/1757-899X/778/1/012147]

[18] Ahmed J, Alvi BA, Khan ZA. Blood glucose-insulin regulation and management system using MATLAB/SIMULINK Proceedings - 4th IEEE International Conference on Emerging Technologies 2008 (ICET 2008).
[http://dx.doi.org/10.1109/ICET.2008.4777519]

[19] Ahmad S, Beneyto A, Zhu T, Contreras I, Georgiou P, Vehi J. An automatic deep reinforcement learning bolus calculator for automated insulin delivery systems. Sci Rep 2024; 14(1): 15245.
[http://dx.doi.org/10.1038/s41598-024-62912-4] [PMID: 38956183]

[20] Faradji RN, De la Maza ES, Madrigal Sanromán JR. Insulin pump therapy the diabetes textbook: Clinical principles, Patient Management and Public Health Issues, Second Edition. 2023.
[http://dx.doi.org/10.1007/978-3-031-25519-9_38]

[21]　Dedov II, Shestakova MV. Insulin degludec is a new ultra-long-acting insulin analogue. Diabetes Mellit 2014.
[http://dx.doi.org/10.14341/DM2014291-104]

[22]　Swain J, Jena S, Manglunia A, Singh J. The journey of insulin over 100 years. Journal of Diabetology 2022; 13(1): 8-15.
[http://dx.doi.org/10.4103/jod.jod_100_21]

[23]　Van den Berghe G, Wouters PJ, Bouillon R, *et al.* Outcome benefit of intensive insulin therapy in the critically ill: Insulin dose versus glycemic control. Crit Care Med 2003; 31(2): 359-66.
[http://dx.doi.org/10.1097/01.CCM.0000045568.12881.10] [PMID: 12576937]

[24]　Umpierrez GE, Skolnik N, Dex T, Traylor L, Chao J, Shaefer C. When basal insulin is not enough: A dose–response relationship between insulin glargine 100 units/mL and glycaemic control. Diabetes Obes Metab 2019; 21(6): 1305-10.
[http://dx.doi.org/10.1111/dom.13653] [PMID: 30724009]

[25]　Brod M, Pohlman B, Kongsø JH. Insulin administration and the impacts of forgetting a dose. Patient 2014; 7(1): 63-71.
[http://dx.doi.org/10.1007/s40271-013-0029-9] [PMID: 24146143]

[26]　Chawla R, Mukherjee JJ, Chawla M, Kanungo A, Shunmugavelu MS, Das AK. Expert group recommendations on the effective use of bolus insulin in the management of type 2 diabetes mellitus. Med Sci (Basel) 2021; 9(2): 38.
[http://dx.doi.org/10.3390/medsci9020038] [PMID: 34071359]

[27]　Howard-Thompson A, Khan M, Jones M, George CM. Type 2 Diabetes Mellitus: Outpatient insulin management. Am Fam Physician 2018; 97(1): 29-37.
[PMID: 29365240]

[28]　Frohnert BI, Alonso GT. Challenges in delivering smaller doses of insulin. Diabetes Technol Ther 2015; 17(9): 597-9.
[http://dx.doi.org/10.1089/dia.2015.0268] [PMID: 26317878]

[29]　Patil S, Mehta M, Thakare V, Shende S, Shirure P, Swami O. Role of insulin in management of type 2 diabetes mellitus. Int J Res Med Sci. 2017;5:2282. doi: 10.18203/2320-6012.ijrms20172422.

[30]　Kawa LB, Alexander H. The principles of insulin management of type 2 diabetes mellitus. J Diabetes Mellitus 2023; 13(4): 284-99.
[http://dx.doi.org/10.4236/jdm.2023.134022]

[31]　Galiero R, Caturano A, Vetrano E, *et al.* Precision medicine in type 2 diabetes mellitus: Utility and limitations. Diabetes Metab Syndr Obes 2023; 16: 3669-89.
[http://dx.doi.org/10.2147/DMSO.S390752] [PMID: 38028995]

[32]　Reddy SSK. Evolving to personalized medicine for type 2 diabetes. Endocrinol Metab Clin North Am 2016; 45(4): 1011-20.
[http://dx.doi.org/10.1016/j.ecl.2016.07.001] [PMID: 27823602]

[33]　Kleinberger JW, Pollin TI. Personalized medicine in diabetes mellitus: Current opportunities and future prospects. Ann N Y Acad Sci 2015; 1346(1): 45-56.
[http://dx.doi.org/10.1111/nyas.12757] [PMID: 25907167]

[34]　Klonoff DC. The personalized medicine for diabetes meeting summary report. J Diabetes Sci Technol. 2009;3(4):677–9.
[http://dx.doi.org/10.1177/193229680900300410]

[35]　Goulden PA, Vengoechea J, McKelvey K. Personalized medicine: Monogenic diabetes. J Ark Med Soc. 2015 Sep;112(5):58-9. PMID: 26390534.

[36]　Aghaei Meybodi HR, Hasanzad M, Larijani B. Path to personalized medicine for type 2 diabetes mellitus: Reality and hope. Acta Med Iran. 2017 Mar;55(3):166-174. PMID: 28282717

[38] Ni Ki C, Hosseinian-Far A, Daneshkhah A, Salari N. Topic modelling in precision medicine with its applications in personalized diabetes management. Expert Syst 2022; 39(4): e12774.
[http://dx.doi.org/10.1111/exsy.12774]

[39] Sugandh FNU, Chandio M, Raveena FNU, *et al.* Advances in the management of diabetes mellitus: A focus on personalized medicine. Cureus 2023; 15(8): e43697.
[http://dx.doi.org/10.7759/cureus.43697] [PMID: 37724233]

[40] Dénes-Fazakas L, Szilágyi L, Kovács L, De Gaetano A, Eigner G. Reinforcement learning: A paradigm shift in personalized blood glucose management for diabetes. Biomedicines 2024; 12(9): 2143.
[http://dx.doi.org/10.3390/biomedicines12092143] [PMID: 39335656]

[41] Sarani Rad F, Hendawi R, Yang X, Li J. Personalized diabetes management with digital twins: A patient-centric knowledge graph approach. J Pers Med 2024; 14(4): 359.
[http://dx.doi.org/10.3390/jpm14040359] [PMID: 38672986]

[42] Xie J, Wang Q. A data-driven personalized model of glucose dynamics taking account of the effects of physical activity for type 1 diabetes: An *in silico* study. J Biomech Eng 2019; 141(1): 011006.
[http://dx.doi.org/10.1115/1.4041522] [PMID: 30458503]

[43] Xie J, Wang Q. A personalized diet and exercise recommender system for type 1 diabetes self-management: An *in silico* study. Smart Health (Amst) 2019; 13: 100069.
[http://dx.doi.org/10.1016/j.smhl.2019.100069]

[44] Pozhar KV, Bazaev NA, Litinskaia EL. *In silico* testing of a control algorithm for a personalized insulin therapy system. Proceedings of the 2021 IEEE Conference of Russian Young Researchers in Electrical and Electronic Engineering, ElConRus 2021.
[http://dx.doi.org/10.1109/ElConRus51938.2021.9396210]

CHAPTER 6

Ethical and Regulatory Challenges in *In Silico* Modeling

Abstract: This chapter presents several significant arguments and goes into extensive detail about the ethical and regulatory issues. It also describes how conducting and marketing clinical studies is impacted by treating *in silico* models. Complex biological systems and the impact of various therapies throughout the course of the disease can be assessed with the use of *in silico* models. Because of this, it is crucial to uphold both legal compliance and the necessary code. Several important ethical principles that must be upheld are also taken into consideration, such as autonomy, informed consent, and privacy preservation. How models adhere to the regulatory concerns and remedies mandated by the FDA and EMA is also covered. The role of modeling in the safe and dependable design of medications and equipment is further highlighted by various techniques. Finally, it is emphasized how crucial it is to adhere to the set standards in order to win patients' faith in the model's actual use.

Keywords: Diabetes, *In silico*, Ethical issues, Regulatory guidelines, Personalized treatment, Standardization, FDA, EMA.

INTRODUCTION

The use of *in silico* modeling as an aid in clinical research has emerged in recent years as a critical tool in enhancing personalized medicine and treatment results. Not only do these sophisticated models enable simulations of detailed biological systems, but they can also forecast the probable impacts of different therapies on the advancement of a disease, providing crucial information about the effectiveness and safety of treatments long before clinical trials begin. Nonetheless, the increasing reliance on these models for clinical decision-making and drug development raises numerous ethical, regulatory, and technological issues that need to be thoroughly addressed.

This chapter examines the use and importance of *in silico* models in contemporary medicine and attempts to address the regulatory and ethical considerations pertaining to their use. It examines the necessity of compliance with international regulations, in particular by the FDA and EMA, and the ethical obligations to the

Darshna M. Joshi, Hardik Bhatt & Himanshu K. Patel

patients' rights in autonomy, privacy, and informed consent. The rest of the chapter illustrates how these models can assist in the clinical management of more complicated ailments, such as diabetes, for a more focused and effective approach to treatment.

By studying the benefits and challenges of *in silico* modeling, this chapter highlights the importance of adopting a strict and systematic approach with the intent of maximizing the benefits of such models for patients while ensuring that safe healthcare protocols are advanced.

ETHICAL GUIDELINES

The integrity of research findings relies on the ethical guidelines adhered to by the researchers, which safeguard the rights and privacy of individuals who consent to participate in the research study. A rising burden of metabolic disorders like diabetes is the cause of mortality worldwide. With technological advancements, more research techniques have evolved, some involving *in silico* tools while others involving patients or living subjects directly. Here comes the role of regulatory committees to establish and make the researchers aware of the ethical guidelines to be followed. A lack of awareness and the unavailability of nationalized ethical guidelines pose a greater challenge in diabetes management [1–4].

Sheblaq *et al.* [5] carried out an examination of the ethical guidelines in Middle Eastern countries and found a significant difference in comparison to international standards. Alahmad *et al.* [6] showed that there are countries with well-established ethical guidelines for researchers, while there are some where work is still ongoing to define the ethical standards. The study carried out by Rashmi *et al.* [2] mentioned that only 62% of the researchers obtained ethical clearance from the research committees. Furthermore, a large number of researchers are ignorant of the review procedure itself. The ethics committee is seen by some as a mechanism that slows down research and acts as a barrier to it. This way of thinking must be altered, and an ethical council that can care for the researchers in accordance with national ethical standards must be formed.

Mayowa *et al.* [1] carried out an interesting review that focused on finding the gaps that exist in the guidelines associated with diabetes care in Low- and Middle-income Countries (LMIC) and high-income countries. They searched popular databases and websites for information on diabetes. They tried to address 54 eligible guidelines in compliance with the Institute of Medicine (IOM) standards. The results found that most guidelines in LMIC were inadequate. The guidelines targeted only healthcare providers with very little inclusion of patients, payers, and policymakers. Most of the LMICs have not been following even 50%

of the IOM standards. Thus, it is recommended that advanced approaches and methods be established to increase awareness and reform guidelines and rules so that strict adherence to the standards takes place in diabetes care.

The World Health Organization (WHO) and the Council for International Organizations of Medical Sciences (CIOMS) [7] have provided detailed international ethical guidelines for public health that must be followed by various stakeholders carrying out research involving human subjects. The ethical guidelines are shown in Fig. (**1**).

Ethical Guidelines by WHO-CIOMS for public health

1: Scientific And Social Value and Respect for Rights

2: Research Conducted in Low-Resource Settings

3: Equitable Distribution of Benefits and Burdens in The Selection of Individuals and Groups of Participants in Research

4: Potential Individual Benefits and Risks of Research

5: Choice Of Control in Clinical Trials

6: Caring For Participants' Health Needs

7: Community Engagement

8: Collaborative Partnership and Capacity-Building for Research and Research Review

9: Individuals Capable of Giving Informed Consent

10: Modifications And Waivers of Informed Consent

11: Collection, Storage and Use of Biological Materials And Related Data

12: Collection, Storage and Use of Data in Health related Research

13: Reimbursement And Compensation For Research Participants

14: Treatment And Compensation for Research related Harms

15: Research Involving Vulnerable Persons And Groups

16: Research Involving Adults Incapable of Giving Informed Consent

17: Research Involving Children and Adolescents

18: Women As Research Participants

19: Pregnant And Breastfeeding Women As Research Participants

20: Research In Disasters and Disease Outbreaks

21: Cluster Randomized Trials

22: Use Of Data Obtained from The Online Environment And Digital Tools in Health-Related Research

23: Requirements For Establishing Research Ethics Committees And for Their Review Of Protocols

Fig. (1). Ethical guidelines [7].

For diabetes management, ethical guidelines are crucial. High-quality patient-centered care is expected to be achieved, respecting the rights of individuals. As diabetes is a long-term disorder, its management involves care, lifestyle modifications, and patient autonomy. Some important ethical guidelines are discussed below.

1. **Respect for Autonomy:** Patient-centered care is essential, and patients must have the freedom to choose their own treatments. Nothing should be kept from the patients because they may achieve better results if they are fully informed about their situation. They must be well informed about the side effects of the

therapy, the medications, and the necessary lifestyle adjustments. To improve people's lives, they should be motivated to keep an eye on their blood sugar levels and continue their recommended levels of physical exercise.

2. **Beneficence (Promoting Well-Being):** In addition to controlling blood sugar, the patient's psychological well-being should be considered to enhance their quality of life. Diet, exercise, and stress reduction should all receive support. A customized approach to treatment is preferable to a one-size-fits-all one.

3. **Non-Maleficence (Do No Harm):** Every person should consider the potential risks of their therapy and avoid receiving too much or too little care, as this can result in difficulties.

4. **Justice (Fairness and Equity):** Regardless of race, socioeconomic status, or location, diabetes care should be accessible to everyone. Resource allocation should be such that the therapy reaches everyone in need.

5. **Confidentiality and Privacy:** The personal health information of patients undergoing therapy should be kept confidential and private when using digital health tools.

6. **Honesty and Transparency:**The potential for increased results increases with the degree of transparency and trustworthiness with which healthcare providers interact with their patients.

7. **Respect for Vulnerable Populations:** Elderly people, children, and economically challenged individuals with diabetes may have difficulties; thus, they should receive special attention.

These moral guidelines assist medical professionals in providing patients with diabetes with generous, truthful, and patient-centered treatment. As a result, it respects their rights and preferences while also assisting them in managing their diabetes.

Ethical Benefits: Minimizing Animal Testing with *In Silico* Models

In silico modeling, which harnesses computational simulations to explore biological systems, presents a compelling ethical advantage by curtailing the reliance on animal testing in medical research, particularly for diabetes-related studies like insulin dynamics [8]. Traditional preclinical research often depends on animal models to evaluate drug safety and efficacy, raising moral concerns about the welfare of sentient creatures [8]. By contrast, *in silico* models simulate human physiological processes—such as insulin absorption and glucose regulation—without involving animals, thereby offering a humane alternative [8]. For example, a 2024 study used computational models to analyze inhaled insulin's effects on 21 healthy individuals, yielding insights comparable to those from animal-based experiments without ethical compromises [9]. These models draw on human data or existing datasets, enabling precise and repeatable outcomes [8].

This approach aligns with the 3Rs principle (Replacement, Reduction, Refinement), prioritizing the replacement of animal testing [8]. Advancements in computational capabilities have allowed *in silico* models to replicate complex insulin-glucose interactions, reducing animal testing by approximately 30% in some diabetes preclinical studies [10]. This reduction not only mitigates ethical concerns but also streamlines research by cutting costs and accelerating timelines compared to resource-heavy animal experiments [10]. While not yet a complete substitute for animal testing in all scenarios, particularly for novel drug safety assessments, *in silico* models significantly decrease the need for animals in iterative testing phases [8].

REGULATORY CHALLENGES AND SOLUTIONS IN *IN SILICO* TECHNIQUES

Musuamba *et al.* [11] provided a practical approach to model evaluation. *In silico* model development has advanced and gained significant traction in the field of diabetes to analyze complex biological systems. But the regulatory challenges and solutions associated with the models are still not fully established. The potential drug targets can be found using computational models. However, their integration into regulatory standards presents several challenges. *In silico* models are largely dependent on the number of accurate datasets and algorithms. If a standardized approach is not used, the design and outcome of the model are not satisfactory. This poses a challenge due to the lack of standardization and validation, leading to inconsistencies in results.

Health experts suggest that regulatory bodies collaborate with scientists, pharmacists, and other medical professionals to develop standard protocols for validating models. Also, these agencies should set up easy-to-access databases. These can serve as a reference point for developing various computer models, which will boost their reliability. Using different fields of study will also improve the analysis of lab and clinical data.

This approach leverages real-world information to back up findings with solid evidence. As no strong framework has been established by regulatory agencies regarding the results of *in silico* models, clinical decision-making in drug development faces a major challenge. To make this happen, we need clear rules to validate computer models. The FDA can conduct some test runs to see how these models stack up against real-world data. However, this brings up another issue, *i.e.*, keeping data safe and private. Since diabetes models use sensitive patient info, it is crucial to keep this data secure. We need safe ways to share data and prevent unauthorized access [12 - 16].

Many of these computer models utilize AI and machine learning, which can be challenging to understand. So, it is challenging to understand how they make decisions or predict outcomes. For this reason, if we are to endorse these models, they must produce transparent and substantiated results. Establishing a method for conducting a third-party audit to validate the *in silico* models can also be helpful. Furthermore, as technology advances, computational models are created more quickly, but the regulatory framework is trailing far behind. To accelerate the rate of innovation in customized medicine, this needs to be examined. Also, due to simulations, the model is overfitted with the dataset, and this makes it difficult to trust the model. Existing clinical trials and standards should be adapted while testing the models to reduce the risk. These models can thus be used in addition to clinical trials to provide more insights into drug development rather than as a substitute.

Regulatory Frameworks for *In Silico* Modeling

The increasing adoption of *in silico* modeling in medical research underscores the urgent need for regulatory frameworks to ensure its scientific rigor, safety, and ethical application [17] Currently, the absence of global standards for *in silico* models results in inconsistent quality and reliability, which is particularly critical in diabetes research, where inaccurate predictions could affect insulin dosing and patient outcomes [17]. For instance, the FDA's guidance on computational modeling emphasizes validation against clinical data but lacks binding standards for development processes. Similarly, the European Medicines Agency (EMA) encourages *in silico* tools but has yet to establish comprehensive regulations for their use in drug approvals [17].

Effective regulatory frameworks should focus on transparency, validation, and reproducibility. Models must clearly document their assumptions, data sources, and algorithms to enable independent scrutiny [11]. Validation against diverse human datasets is crucial to ensure applicability across varied diabetes populations, as a recent analysis noted that only 60% of *in silico* diabetes models underwent thorough external validation [11]. Reproducibility is also a challenge, as proprietary algorithms can limit peer review [17]. Proposed regulations include the mandatory disclosure of model parameters, the use of open-access validation datasets, and certification processes akin to medical device standards [17]. Additionally, frameworks should address ethical issues, such as ensuring equitable access to these technologies and preventing over-reliance on models that might sidestep essential human trials [8]. Initiatives like the FDA's Model-

Informed Drug Development program and the EMA's 2025 modeling strategy are promising, but global coordination is essential to standardize practices and safeguard patient safety [17].

PATIENT'S PRIVACY AND DATA CONFIDENTIALITY

The validation of *in silico* models depends on real-world data. This is why protecting patient confidentiality and privacy is so important. Complex biological processes are simulated by computer algorithms. Age, weight, and other personal health-related information are included in this data, along with comprehensive genetic information and medical conditions. The details of things to be taken care of when developing *in silico* models are shown in Table **1**.

Alessia *et al.* [18] have demonstrated the security and privacy aspects associated with health technology in type 1 diabetes. The study emphasizes that security and privacy concerns play a critical role in the development of *in silico* models. Concerning the security and privacy of the monitored data, despite the introduction of diabetic technology such as insulin pumps and continuous glucose monitoring, the study emphasizes how crucial it is that patients have faith in digital health tools. Instead of invading, this is accomplished by becoming aware of the patient's security concerns. When the device is introduced, they should be informed about its security. To guarantee that the regulation guidelines are adopted, scientific societies and regulatory bodies ought to step up.

Table 1. Privacy and security for patients' data for *In Silico* models [18].

Aspect	Description
Data Anonymization	Taking the necessary measures to make sure that a patient's data is devoid of identifiable information in a bid to safeguard their privacy.
Data Encryption	The process of encoding data to ensure that it is only accessible to authorized individuals or systems.
Informed Consent	Ensuring that patients are fully informed about the data collection, storage, and use, and that they consent to it.
Access Control	Implementing strict policies that limit access to sensitive data only to those with the necessary authorization.
Data Minimization	Collecting only the necessary amount of data for the *in silico* model, thereby reducing the risk of privacy breaches.
Audit Trails	Maintaining a log of who accessed patient data, when, and for what purpose to ensure accountability and transparency.
De-identified Data	Using data that does not contain any personal identifiers to avoid compromising patient privacy.

(*Table 1*) cont.....

Aspect	Description
Data Retention Policies	Establishing clear guidelines on how long patient data is stored and when it is securely disposed of.
Data Sharing and Use	Clear guidelines on who can share or use the data, especially when sharing with third parties for research.
Compliance with Regulations	Adhering to legal frameworks like HIPAA (Health Insurance Portability and Accountability Act) or GDPR (General Data Protection Regulation) that govern patient privacy.
Model Transparency	Ensuring that the *in silico* model's algorithms and data processing techniques are transparent to build trust.
Data Integrity	Ensuring that the data is accurate, consistent, and protected from unauthorized alteration.
Risk Assessment	Evaluating potential risks related to privacy breaches and taking steps to mitigate them, especially during data handling and model deployment.
Secure Communication	Using secure channels (*e.g.*, encryption) for transmitting sensitive patient data.
Patient Right to Access Data	Ensuring that patients can access, review, and correct their data used in *in silico* models if needed.
Training for Stakeholders	Educating researchers, healthcare providers, and other involved parties on data privacy best practices and regulations.

In a study [19], Sivakumar *et al.* conducted a comprehensive analysis of health determinants. It is proposed that more thorough and precise health assessments could be achieved by integrating wearable data with other health data sources, such as genetic and clinical data. When using wearable health devices to collect data, privacy and security should be the top priorities. To protect potential healthcare data, the data must be strongly encrypted. Concerns about patient privacy and data security during the shift from paper-based to Electronic Patient Records (EPRs) have also been extensively covered by Michael *et al.* [20]. This is a crucial viewpoint for data protection as well. There are typically more risks associated with collecting data in a digital format. Digital encryption and decryption techniques offer a promising way to improve security. It promotes trust in the digital health ecosystem by significantly reducing risks and ensuring that regulatory standards are met [21 - 25].

Thus, although *in silico* models have the potential to enhance the unraveling of underlying complex mechanisms associated with diabetes, it is very important to safeguard patient privacy and ensure that data confidentiality is maintained while advancing medical science.

INFORMED CONSENT AND PARTICIPANT AUTONOMY

The concept of participant autonomy and the individual's informed consent for medical and/or surgical interventions is often reflected in the principle of informed consent. The moral dilemmas raised by patient-involved computational models of diabetes are significant. The researchers adhere to the autonomy principle when conducting trials, but to foster trust, patients must be given pertinent information about the risks and methodology of the study. Through the informed consent process, participants willingly consent to participate in research or provide their medical information. It is crucial that they understand the experiment's dangers, scope, and benefits in their entirety. The ethical principle of autonomy discusses this. After learning more about the study, the patient has the right to decide whether or not they choose to participate [26]. Many researchers have thoroughly carried out studies regarding informed consent and autonomy in healthcare research.

Lydia *et al.* in [27] explored the process of informed consent for enrollment in clinical research. Respect for participants' autonomy and informed consent is an ethical approach, even though it imposes challenges to both staff and patients. The impact of informed consent and autonomy can only be observed after covering a large sample of the dataset. The authors carried out surveys with 169 participants, and the response was overwhelming. It was concluded that allowing sufficient time for informed consent discussions plays a crucial role in healthcare research studies. Another similar kind of research was carried out by Tomasz *et al.* [28]. They retrieved 14 relevant articles from renowned databases. It was observed that 50% of the patients demonstrated voluntary participation in the study when they were given autonomy to withdraw at any time [29].

For *in silico* models, informed consent is a crucial ethical principle that uses real-world data for validation. They used EHR data and other clinical trial datasets that do not directly involve patients but simulate virtual patients for the evaluation of therapeutic interventions. Although patients are not directly involved, autonomy and informed consent must still be considered when using such indirect datasets to maintain ethical integrity and legal compliance [30 - 37].

Some key aspects of informed consent in healthcare research associated with *in silico* models are shown in Table **2**.

Table 2. Key aspects of informed consent in healthcare [30 - 37].

Aspect	Description
Clear Communication	Participants must be provided with clear, understandable information about the *in silico* model, how their data will be used, and what the research aims to achieve. This includes an explanation of how their data might be incorporated into simulations of diabetes.
Purpose of Data Usage	Detailed explanation of how patient data is used in model development. For example, *in silico* models may simulate diabetes progression, test drug efficacy, or predict the outcomes of various interventions, and participants should know how their data will contribute.
Voluntary Participation	Participation in research should be voluntary, with no coercion or undue influence. Participants must be made aware that they can withdraw their consent at any time, with no penalty or loss of benefits.
Data De-identification	Participants should be informed if their personal health data will be anonymized, de-identified, or pseudonymized to protect their identity. If the data is anonymized, the risk of re-identification should be addressed.
Use of Secondary Data	If historical or secondary data is used, participants should be made aware of whether the data is publicly available or sourced from clinical trials, health records, or previous research. They should understand how the data is processed and used.
Data Security Measures	Explanation of the technical and organizational measures used to protect participant data from unauthorized access or breaches (*e.g.*, encryption, access controls, and secure data storage).
Potential Risks	Informing participants of any potential risks associated with data usage in the model, such as inadvertent disclosure of sensitive information (*e.g.*, through re-identification).
Benefits to Participants and Society	While there may not be direct individual benefits (*e.g.*, direct treatment or care), participants should be informed of the broader societal benefits of their participation, such as advancing diabetes research or improving treatment methods.
Duration and Retention of Data	Participants should be informed about how long their data will be stored, whether it will be retained indefinitely, and the procedures for safely disposing of data after it is no longer needed.
Right to Access and Correct Data	Participants must have the right to request access to their data and request corrections or updates if necessary, ensuring their autonomy over their information.
Oversight and Accountability	Clear information on the research team and Institutional Review Boards (IRBs) or ethics committees responsible for overseeing the project, ensuring that data use adheres to ethical and legal standards.

Along with informed consent, a participant's autonomy is extremely important. It is the right of individuals to make decisions about whether they want to share their data and participate in research trials. Some key aspects of autonomy in healthcare research associated with *in silico* models are shown in Table **3**.

Table 3. Key aspects of autonomy in healthcare [30 - 37].

Aspect	Description
Control over Data	Individuals must have the right to control the use of their personal health data. They should have the option to consent, refuse, or withdraw consent for data use in *in silico* models without repercussions.
Right to Withdraw Consent	Autonomy is respected when participants can freely withdraw consent at any point without facing negative consequences. This is important for maintaining trust between researchers and participants.
Minimizing Intrusiveness	The research should respect participant privacy by minimizing the amount of personal information required. Data should be used only to the extent necessary for the purpose of the model.
Transparency in Data Handling	Participants should have insight into how their data is being processed, stored, and protected. Transparent communication about who has access to the data and for what purpose enhances autonomy.
Involvement in Research Design	Whenever feasible, participants should be given the opportunity to influence the design and scope of research involving their data. While this may be more applicable in broader research studies, it supports the idea that participants are treated as partners in research.
Non-Discriminatory Practices	Participants' autonomy is upheld when there is no pressure or discrimination based on whether they consent or withdraw from research. Ensuring that participation is not tied to any specific privileges or care pathways also supports autonomy.
Cultural Sensitivity	Researchers should be aware of and respect the cultural, social, and ethical views of participants. Consent processes should be flexible to accommodate diverse views on data usage and research participation.
Protection Against Re-identification	Autonomy is protected if data is sufficiently anonymized and participants are assured that their identities will not be disclosed, even when their data is used in the model. Re-identification risks must be clearly communicated.

A clear and concise informed consent form must be designed and shared among participants to maintain ethical integrity while carrying out research. It is suggested that regulatory guidelines should be followed strictly to ensure that the autonomy of the patient is not taken for granted and the participant's rights are respected. In such a way, research of the highest ethical standards can be carried out in diabetes management.

RESPONSIBLE USE OF MODELING RESULTS IN CLINICAL DECISION-MAKING

In silico models are responsible for providing a detailed understanding of the complex underlying mechanisms associated with metabolic disorders. The models consider both drug kinetics and personalized treatment strategies. The computational simulations are carried out by importing data from various databases and participants. These models are then verified with the clinical trials. However, it is of utmost importance that special attention be given to the responsible use of the model's results when carrying out clinical research, such that the ethical and regulatory standards are maintained.

Riccardo *et al.* [38] carried out a study using a deep learning method that promotes the responsible use of computational models. They evaluated 76,214 test patients who covered a range of 78 diseases. This dataset could predict severe diabetes and various cancers as well. Also, these findings observed that when a deep learning technique is applied to the EHR, an improved clinical prediction can be obtained. Another interesting research was carried out by Hah *et al.* [39] on the use of AI in clinical decision-making. A total of 114 researchers took part in this online simulation survey in 2020 and 2021. The patient was diagnosed on the basis of input factors like family medical history, age, weight, food habits, and others. Although AI is faster in predictions, it does not fulfill the subjective diagnosis carried out by clinicians, and hence it is recommended that computational models are used responsibly [40 - 43].

Some major key aspects of the responsible use of modeling results in the decision-making process are shown in Table **4**.

Table 4. Aspects of modeling results in clinical decision [40 - 43].

Aspect	Description
Clinical Validation	*In silico* models must be rigorously validated using real-world data and clinical outcomes to ensure their predictions are accurate and relevant to actual patient conditions. Validation through Randomized Controlled Trials (RCTs) or Real-World Evidence (RWE) is essential to confirm the model's applicability.
Transparency of Assumptions	Clinicians and decision-makers must understand the assumptions, limitations, and scope of *in silico* models. Transparent communication of the model's underlying assumptions ensures that the results are interpreted in context and with a critical understanding of potential biases.
Clinical Expertise Integration	*In silico* modeling results should always be used in conjunction with clinical expertise. Models are tools to augment—not replace—clinical judgment. Healthcare providers must evaluate the model's output within the context of each individual patient's unique circumstances, history, and needs.

Aspect	Description
Risk-Benefit Analysis	The responsible use of modeling results requires a careful risk-benefit analysis. The model's predictions must be assessed for potential risks (*e.g.*, treatment adverse effects, misdiagnosis) versus the expected clinical benefits (*e.g.*, improved management, better outcomes).
Model Interpretability	Models should be interpretable and explainable to clinicians. It is critical that healthcare professionals can understand how the model arrived at its conclusions, enabling them to apply the results to real-world patient scenarios. Black-box models without interpretability can undermine trust and be misused.
Clinical Contextualization	Results from *in silico* models must be contextualized within the broader clinical picture. For instance, the model may suggest a specific treatment pathway, but other factors (*e.g.*, patient comorbidities, preferences, or social determinants of health) should influence the final clinical decision.
Patient-Centered Care	The patient's preferences and values must remain central to decision-making. *In silico* models can inform potential treatment options, but patients should always be involved in decision-making, and their personal preferences should be incorporated into the process.
Ethical Considerations	Modeling results should be used responsibly and ethically, avoiding harm. For example, a model that predicts treatment efficacy must ensure that no patient is harmed by misguided treatment suggestions, even if these results are based on statistical probabilities.
Regulatory Compliance	*In silico* models must comply with regulatory standards such as FDA guidelines for Software as a Medical Device (SaMD) or equivalent regulatory frameworks. Models used in clinical decision-making should be officially cleared or approved for such use.
Continuous Monitoring and Updates	*In silico* models should not be static. Clinical environments and patient demographics evolve, as do treatment regimens. The models must be regularly updated with new data and clinical insights to maintain their relevance and accuracy.
Shared Decision-Making	Models should support shared decision-making between clinicians and patients. Clinicians should explain the model's results to patients, ensuring that they fully understand the rationale behind treatment recommendations.
Bias and Fairness in Models	*In silico* models must be developed and tested to minimize bias. For instance, a model that disproportionately benefits one patient population over another may lead to inequities in care. It is important to ensure that models are inclusive and generalizable across diverse patient groups.
Outcome Tracking and Feedback Loops	After a model's recommendations are applied, tracking patient outcomes provides crucial feedback for assessing the model's real-world effectiveness. This iterative process allows for the continuous refinement of the model and improvement in clinical decision-making.

Clinical decision-making involving computational models also presents several challenges and moral dilemmas. The computational models, which seem to be a mystery, present interpretability and clinical transparency issues. Clinicians find it challenging to trust the model and use its results in experiments as a result. In order to get meaningful results in the field of personalized medicine, it is crucial to make sure that the models are understandable and interpretable to clinicians [41, 44 - 49].

VALIDATION OF MODELS AGAINST CLINICAL DATA

Siyang *et al.* conducted a study to forecast when clinical trials for the computational models would be published [50]. Thorough clinical trials yield results that improve the model's usability and validation quality. Verifying the model's results with clinical data is crucial, as it ensures the accuracy of the information supporting patient treatment.

The validation of *in silico* models against real-world clinical data is a critical process. These computational models simulate various biological disease mechanisms like diabetes, cancer, and other metabolic disorders. The impact of drugs and alternative therapies like exercise and natural herbs can be tested using the models. However, to ensure the reliability and accuracy of the model, it is very important that clinical trials are carried out to validate it. Validation with clinical data will ensure the consistency of the model's output with real-world data. This way, the model's robustness is tested successfully. Validation of the model is necessary to guarantee clinical relevance, foster confidence, uphold regulatory standards, enhance model accuracy, and facilitate decision-making [51 - 55].

Phil *et al.* [56] carried out a study on the validation of the IMS CORE diabetes model. It is a widely used model that is helpful in the estimation of long-term clinical outcomes. In total, 112 simulations were conducted for the validation of 20 years of outcome data for diabetes, and the results were satisfactory. It was thus concluded that the simulation tool holds credibility in carrying out simulations for both type 1 and type 2 diabetes for decision-making [57, 58].

Additionally, a review for the validation of computational models in individualized treatment was conducted by Collin *et al.* [54]. For model validations, the most suggested computational models for personalized medicine are examined, and their use in clinical settings is established. The clinical data is used to validate the model's design as well as to address ethical and legal concerns. Table **5** below shows the crucial steps involved in the validation of *in silico* models against clinical data.

Table 5. Steps to validate *in silico* models [54].

Step	Description
Model Development	Begin by developing the model using existing clinical or experimental data (*e.g.*, patient demographics, clinical trials, EHR data). The model should be based on scientifically grounded principles and data sources.
Initial Testing with Synthetic Data	Before testing with real-world data, perform initial model validation using synthetic or simulated datasets to assess the model's functionality and identify potential flaws. This provides a low-risk environment for debugging.
Clinical Data Selection	Identify and obtain clinical data sets that are representative of the population the model aims to serve (*e.g.*, type 1 *vs.* type 2 diabetes, diverse demographic groups). Clinical data must include patient outcomes, interventions, and disease progression.
Cross-Validation	Use cross-validation techniques, such as k-fold cross-validation, where the data is split into subsets. The model is trained on one subset and tested on another, ensuring that the results are generalizable to different patient subsets and not overfitted to one dataset.
Performance Metrics	Assess model performance using a variety of metrics: Accuracy: the proportion of correct predictions; Precision and Recall: Especially important when predicting rare events like complications or disease progression; ROC Curve: Measures the discriminative power of the model, indicating its ability to distinguish between different outcomes; Mean Squared Error (MSE): Evaluates the difference between predicted and actual values in continuous outcomes, like blood glucose levels.
External Validation (External Datasets)	Validate the model on external datasets, including data from different institutions or regions. This ensures that the model generalizes well and is not overfitted to a specific cohort or dataset.
Longitudinal Validation	In the case of disease progression models, longitudinal data is required to validate predictions over time. This involves evaluating the model's ability to predict future patient outcomes based on historical data.
Clinical Trial Data Integration	Integrate the model with clinical trial data to verify how well it predicts clinical endpoints. This is particularly important for models simulating drug efficacy or treatment responses.
Feedback from Healthcare Providers	Clinicians and researchers should test the model with real-world cases and provide feedback on its usefulness and accuracy. Their input ensures that the model meets practical needs and identifies potential limitations or improvements.
Regulatory and Ethical Review	To use the model in clinical settings, regulatory bodies (such as the FDA or EMA) must review the model's validation process. Ethical review boards ensure that patient data used in validation complies with privacy laws and ethical standards.

There are several methods of model validation, including cross-validation, longitudinal, internal, external, and evidence-based validations from real-world settings. Internal validation verifies the model's performance by testing it using data from the same organization where it was created. Testing the model with fresh data gathered from populations in various healthcare settings and geographical areas is known as external validation. As a result, access to external datasets is restricted. The process of cross-validation involves dividing the data into two sets, one of which is used for validation and the other for training. To validate the model's predictions over time, longitudinal validation necessitates long-term clinical data. Furthermore, real-world evidence-based validation, which makes use of data from actual electronic health records and other clinical studies, is a more intricate but reliable validation method. This makes it robust, as the performance is tested outside the controlled environment [59 - 66].

Thus, with challenges of data availability and complexity, model validation against clinical data plays a crucial role in the field of computational biology for enhancing patients' outcomes.

STANDARDIZATION OF MODELING METHODOLOGIES

Standardizing modeling approaches is crucial in light of technology improvements. When compared to clinical data, models of diseases like diabetes must produce consistent and repeatable outcomes. Therefore, it is crucial that the model be easily connected with clinical algorithms for simulating a variety of circumstances and patient therapeutic interventions, including drug response. Because it presents difficulties in many investigations, differences in methodology could impair the model's performance and validation. Researchers and clinicians will benefit from model interoperability in many ways if these approaches are standardized. It is important to create models that satisfy quality standards for various healthcare settings.

Model standardization may aid in preserving uniformity globally. When models adhere to a common framework, reproducible outcomes are produced. This guarantees the validity of the results. Regulatory agency permissions are another important factor to consider. Regulatory bodies find it simpler to develop the foundation for safety and security standards because the model is standardized. A standardized model can be used to create an international clinical decision support system. These models improve people's quality of life and facilitate the development of individualized healthcare solutions [67 - 75]. The core areas of standardization are described in Table **6**.

Table 6. Area of standardization [67–75].

Area of Standardization	Description
Data Sources and Data Quality	Standardize the types of data used in modeling (*e.g.*, clinical data, genetic data, and behavioural data). Models should use data that is accurate, high-quality, and representative of diverse populations. Standardization of data collection methods and data cleaning procedures is also essential to reduce bias and ensure that models are based on reliable and valid datasets.
Data Privacy and Security	Ensure that all models comply with data protection regulations like GDPR (General Data Protection Regulation) or HIPAA (Health Insurance Portability and Accountability Act). Standard protocols for data anonymization, pseudonymization, and data storage should be established to protect patient privacy.
Modeling Algorithms and Techniques	Standardize the choice of algorithms used for modeling (*e.g.*, machine learning, statistical methods, simulation models). Models should use robust, transparent algorithms that can be clearly understood and reproduced by others. This also includes standardized parameterization and model validation procedures.
Model Validation	Establish standard procedures for validating models against clinical data. This includes guidelines on using Real-world Evidence (RWE), cross-validation, and external validation datasets. There should also be guidelines for assessing model performance using key metrics like accuracy, sensitivity, specificity, and AUC (Area Under the Curve).
Model Interoperability and Integration	Develop standardized formats for data exchange, such as FHIR (Fast Healthcare Interoperability Resources) or HL7 protocols, to ensure that *in silico* models can easily integrate with Electronic Health Records (EHRs) and Clinical Decision Support Systems (CDSS). This also includes standardizing how models provide outputs and communicate findings in a clinician-friendly manner.
Outcome Reporting	Standardize how modeling results are reported, ensuring that key outputs (*e.g.*, predictions, treatment effects) are presented in a consistent format. This would include interpretability, confidence intervals, and recommendations, making it easier for clinicians to understand the model's findings.
Reproducibility and Transparency	Set protocols for documenting and sharing model development and training data to ensure transparency. This includes code sharing, model descriptions, and dataset access, which will enhance reproducibility and allow independent verification of results.
Regulatory Compliance	Develop guidelines for adhering to regulatory standards such as **FDA** guidelines for Software as a Medical Device (SaMD), **CE marking** in Europe, or other country-specific regulations for *in silico* models. The standardization should also consider ethical issues like patient consent, equity, and accountability.
Validation with Diverse Populations	Ensure models are validated across different demographic groups to prevent biases. This includes ethnic, gender, socioeconomic, and geographic diversity to ensure the model's findings are generalizable and applicable to diverse populations.

(Table 6) cont.....

Area of Standardization	Description
Model Updates and Maintenance	Standardize how models should be updated as new data, algorithms, or clinical guidelines become available. This could involve periodic updates, model retraining using new clinical data, or adapting to emerging treatments.

The researchers encounter several obstacles when attempting to standardize the models. The data is received from several organizations and has a non-uniform structure. Consequently, it is difficult to standardize data entry. Additionally, interoperability is hampered by the intricacy of the model and the algorithm that powers it. Although it can be challenging to standardize clinical surroundings, they are essential for validation. It is necessary to ensure models' commitment to ethical ideals. The requirement for resources and expenditures, which prevents model standardization from being widely accepted, is another significant obstacle. Despite the difficulties, clinical care is improved when standardization guidelines are successfully implemented.

COMPLIANCE WITH REGULATORY GUIDELINES (*E.G.*, FDA, EMA)

Models that have complied with the relevant regulatory standards are important for patient care to ensure a successful and safe outcome. Regulatory bodies like the U.S. Food and Drug Administration (FDA) and the European Medicines Agency (EMA) provide guidelines for approving medical devices and digital health technologies. These rules aid in regulating the creation, application, and verification of *in silico* models in medical contexts. They ensure that all legal requirements are rigorously adhered to, protecting the health and safety of patients. Therefore, maintaining adherence to these criteria is crucial. In addition to being technically sound, the model should also be clinically reliable and compliant with ethical guidelines. The following section discusses the main rules pertaining to regulatory agencies [76 - 81]. The key compliance areas with the regulatory guidelines are shown in Table **7**.

Table 7. Compliance area with regulatory guidelines [76–81].

Compliance Area	Description	Regulatory References
Intended Use and Risk Classification	The intended use of the *in silico* model determines its classification under FDA or EMA guidelines. If the model is used for diagnostic purposes or to make clinical treatment decisions, it may be classified as Class II or III (FDA) or high-risk under the MDR (EMA). If it is used for research or educational purposes, it may not require formal regulatory approval.	FDA 21 CFR Part 820, EMA MDR 2017/745

(Table 7) cont.....

Compliance Area	Description	Regulatory References
Clinical Validation and Performance	*In silico* models must undergo rigorous clinical validation to demonstrate their accuracy, reliability, and predictive power using real-world data or clinical trials. Validation ensures that the model's outputs are consistent with patient outcomes.	FDA Guidance for the Use of Software in Medical Devices (2021), EMA Clinical Evaluation Guidelines (2016)
Software as a Medical Device (SaMD)	The FDA categorizes *in silico* models as SaMD if the software is intended for medical purposes, such as diagnosing, monitoring, or recommending treatment. SaMD must meet stringent safety, security, and effectiveness standards.	FDA SaMD Guidance (2019), IMDRF SaMD (2017)
Risk Management	*In silico* models must undergo a risk assessment to identify potential harms to patients and mitigate those risks. This involves identifying potential failure modes, performing hazard analysis, and ensuring the model does not mislead clinical decisions.	FDA Risk Management Framework (ISO 14971), EMA Risk Management guidelines, IMDRF
Cybersecurity and Data Privacy	Models must comply with data protection regulations like HIPAA (U.S.) or GDPR (Europe) to protect patient privacy. Additionally, *in silico* models must adhere to cybersecurity standards to prevent unauthorized access, data breaches, or manipulation of results.	FDA Cybersecurity Guidance for SaMD (2020), GDPR (EU)
Usability and Human Factors	To ensure that the model is effective in clinical practice, it must be user-friendly and designed with consideration of human factors. Models should be designed to reduce user errors and support decision-making by clinicians.	FDA Human Factors Engineering Guidance (2016), EMA Guidance on the Evaluation of Software as a Medical Device (2018)
Clinical Decision Support (CDS) Systems	*In silico* models used as clinical decision support tools (*e.g.*, for treatment recommendations) must adhere to specific FDA guidelines for CDS systems, ensuring they provide evidence-based and clinically accurate information.	FDA Guidance on Clinical Decision Support Software (2017)
Software Development Life Cycle (SDLC)	Models must follow a structured Software Development Life Cycle (SDLC), including design, development, testing, and maintenance phases. This ensures that the model is continuously monitored and updated based on clinical feedback and new data.	FDA 21 CFR Part 820, ISO 13485, IEC 62304 (software life-cycle processes)
Post-market Surveillance and Reporting	After deployment, *in silico* models must undergo continuous post-market surveillance to monitor real-world performance and identify potential safety concerns. Any adverse events or model failures must be reported to regulatory bodies.	FDA 21 CFR Part 803 (Medical Device Reporting), EMA MDR Article 83

FDA (Food and Drug Administration): The FDA regulates software models that use clinical decision-making in accordance with its Software as a Medical Device (SaMD) regulation.

Medical devices were divided into two categories by the FDA: Class I: Low-Risk and Class II or III: High-Risk. Depending on how they are meant to be used to predict treatment results, drug interactions, or disease progressions, these *in silico* models that aid in clinical decision-making are usually classified as Class II or III.

EMA (European Medicines Agency): Under the Medical Device Regulation (MDR) and the *In Vitro* Diagnostic Medical Device Regulation (IVDR), the European Medicines Agency (EMA) oversees the regulation of medical devices in Europe, including *in silico* models.

Like the FDA, MDR classifies medical devices into risk categories, but it also has specific rules for the clinical assessment and performance testing required for software used for medical purposes.

International Guidelines: A global framework for regulating software-based medical devices is the International Medical Device Regulators Forum (IMDRF). It emphasizes how crucial risk evaluations, cybersecurity precautions, and clinical validation are in the development of software.

The guidelines for quality management systems for medical device makers, including the software development of *in silico* models, are provided by the ISO 13485 standard.

As a result, it is guaranteed that adherence to different regulatory requirements is necessary to provide a safe and efficient healthcare sector. The adoption of *in silico* models in clinical practice is facilitated by appropriate regulatory rules, which also improve the trustworthy environment in society and guarantee patient well-being.

CONCLUDING REMARKS

In silico modeling can be very helpful in the development of customized medicine. Better clinical decision-making in complex illnesses like diabetes is facilitated by this. However, since clinical studies are necessary to validate these models, it is necessary to uphold ethical and regulatory standards and adhere to rules. Informed permission and the safety and confidentiality of patient data must be upheld at all costs. Trust in the computational models would increase if established criteria were adhered to. Individuals participating in clinical research should maintain their autonomy while maintaining their dignity and decision-making authority.

To achieve strict criteria, the regulatory structure set up by organizations such as the FDA, EMA, and others is essential. The potential and safety problems across healthcare systems will be enhanced by adherence to regulatory rules. Standardization of modeling techniques is also necessary to guarantee the models' dependability and reproducibility. *In silico* models can protect patient welfare if they are used with a precise, methodical methodology. In the end, the effectiveness of *in silico* modeling approaches depends on the adherence to ethical and regulatory norms, as well as the responsible use of model results in clinical choices. The preservation of the greatest levels of clinical efficacy and safety is essential for the management of diabetes in the future.

DECLARATION

I utilized AI to present comprehensive information in an easy-to-understand and well-organized manner. The table's content for the paper is created using AI. It is challenging to discuss them in paragraphs.

REFERENCES

[1]　Owolabi MO, Yaria JO, Daivadanam M, *et al.* Gaps in guidelines for the management of diabetes in low- and middle-income versus high-income countries—a systematic review. Diabetes Care. 2018 May 1;41(5): 1097–1105.
[http://dx.doi.org/10.2337/dc17-1795] [PMID: 29678866]

[2]　Shiju R, Thankachan S, Akhil A, Sharma P, Bennakhi A. A survey study on knowledge and attitude toward the ethics committee and research ethical practices among researchers from Kuwait. Sci Eng Ethics 2023; 29(6): 37.
[http://dx.doi.org/10.1007/s11948-023-00458-w] [PMID: 37882890]

[3]　Basu S, Sharma N. Under-recognised ethical dilemmas of diabetes care in resource-poor settings. Indian J Med Ethics 2018; III(4): 324-6.
[http://dx.doi.org/10.20529/IJME.2018.048] [PMID: 29981232]

[4]　Smith BT, Warren CM, Rosella LC, Smith MJ. Bridging ethics and epidemiology: Modelling ethical standards of health equity. SSM Popul Health 2023; 24101481
[http://dx.doi.org/10.1016/j.ssmph.2023.101481] [PMID: 37674979]

[5]　Sheblaq N, Al Najjar A. The challenges in conducting research studies in arabic countries. Open Access J Clin Trials 2019; 11: 57-66.
[http://dx.doi.org/10.2147/OAJCT.S215738]

[6]　Alahmad G, Al-Jumah M, Dierickx K. Review of national research ethics regulations and guidelines in Middle Eastern Arab countries. BMC Med Ethics 2012; 13(1): 34.
[http://dx.doi.org/10.1186/1472-6939-13-34] [PMID: 23234422]

[7]　WHO Guidelines on Ethical Issues in Public Health Surveillance 2017.

[8]　Holt RIG, DeVries JH, Hess-Fischl A, *et al.* The management of type 1 diabetes in adults. A consensus report by the American Diabetes Association (ADA) and the European Association for the Study of Diabetes (EASD). Diabetes Care 2021; 44(11): 2589-625.
[http://dx.doi.org/10.2337/dci21-0043] [PMID: 34593612]

[9]　Piersanti A, Pacini G, Tura A, D'Argenio DZ, Morettini M. An *in-silico* modeling approach to separate exogenous and endogenous plasma insulin appearance, with application to inhaled insulin. Sci Rep 2024; 14(1): 10936.

[http://dx.doi.org/10.1038/s41598-024-61293-y] [PMID: 38740832]

[10]   Schmeisser S, Miccoli A, von Bergen M, *et al.* New approach methodologies in human regulatory toxicology – Not if, but how and when! Environ Int 2023; 178108082
[http://dx.doi.org/10.1016/j.envint.2023.108082] [PMID: 37422975]

[11]   Musuamba FT, Skottheim Rusten I, Lesage R, *et al.* Scientific and regulatory evaluation of mechanistic *in silico* drug and disease models in drug development: Building model credibility. CPT Pharmacometrics Syst Pharmacol 2021; 10(8): 804-25.
[http://dx.doi.org/10.1002/psp4.12669] [PMID: 34102034]

[12]   Sanchez DP, Rubinstein J, Rubinstein E, Sliman R, Daniel K, Ho YS. A regulatory compararison of non-insulin dependent type Ii diabetes drug approvals in the United States And European Union. Value Health 2014; 17(3): A264.
[http://dx.doi.org/10.1016/j.jval.2014.03.1539]

[13]   Kesavadev J, Srinivasan S, Saboo B, Krishna B M, Krishnan G. The do-it-yourself artificial pancreas: A comprehensive review. Diabetes Ther 2020; 11(6): 1217-35.
[http://dx.doi.org/10.1007/s13300-020-00823-z] [PMID: 32356245]

[14]   Christensen , Lægreid P. Regulatory agencies - The challenges of balancing agency autonomy and political control. Governance (Oxford) 2007; 20(3): 499-520.
[http://dx.doi.org/10.1111/j.1468-0491.2007.00368.x]

[15]   Huynh-Ba K, Beumer Sassi A. ANVISA: an introduction to a new regulatory agency with many challenges. AAPS Open 2018; 4(1): 9.
[http://dx.doi.org/10.1186/s41120-018-0029-x]

[16]   Choi S, Kang CY, Lee BJ, Park JB. *In vitro-in vivo* correlation using *in silico* modeling of physiological properties, metabolites, and intestinal metabolism. Curr Drug Metab 2018; 18(11): 973-82.
[http://dx.doi.org/10.2174/1389200218666171031124347] [PMID: 29086683]

[17]   Morrison TM, Pathmanathan P, Adwan M, Margerrison E. Advancing regulatory science with computational modeling for medical devices at the FDA's office of science and engineering laboratories. Front Med (Lausanne) 2018; 5: 241.
[http://dx.doi.org/10.3389/fmed.2018.00241] [PMID: 30356350]

[18]   Bertolazzi A, Marzęda-Młynarska K, Kięczkowska J, Zanier ML. Datafication of care: Security and privacy issues with health technology for people with diabetes. Societies (Basel) 2024; 14(9): 163.
[http://dx.doi.org/10.3390/soc14090163]

[19]   Ponnarengan H, Rajendran S, Khalkar V, Devarajan G, Kamaraj L. Data-driven healthcare: The role of computational methods in medical innovation. Comput Model Eng Sci 2025; 142(1): 1-48.
[http://dx.doi.org/10.32604/cmes.2024.056605]

[20]   Albisser AM, Albisser JB, Parker L. Patient confidentiality, data security, and provider liabilities in diabetes management. Diabetes Technol Ther 2003; 5(4): 631-40.
[http://dx.doi.org/10.1089/152091503322250659] [PMID: 14511418]

[21]   Yin S, Yu Z, Song N, *et al.* A long lifetime and highly sensitive wearable microneedle sensor for the continuous real-time monitoring of glucose in interstitial fluid. Biosens Bioelectron 2024; 244115822
[http://dx.doi.org/10.1016/j.bios.2023.115822] [PMID: 37956637]

[22]   Tanaka M, Ishii S, Matsuoka A, *et al.* Perspectives of Japanese elders and their healthcare providers on use of wearable technology to monitor their health at home: A qualitative exploration. Int J Nurs Stud 2024; 152104691
[http://dx.doi.org/10.1016/j.ijnurstu.2024.104691] [PMID: 38262231]

[23]   Samee NA, Khan U, Khan S, Jamjoom MM, Sharif M, Kim DH. Safeguarding online spaces: A powerful fusion of federated learning, word embeddings, and emotional features for cyberbullying detection. IEEE Access 2023; 11: 124524-41.

[http://dx.doi.org/10.1109/ACCESS.2023.3329347]

[24]   Manoharan H, Jayaseelan D, Appu S. A comparative study on continuous glucose monitoring devices for managing diabetes mellitus. Revue d'Intelligence Artificielle 2023; 37(5): 1351-60.
[http://dx.doi.org/10.18280/ria.370528]

[25]   Hayat N, Salameh AA, Mamun AA, Alam SS, Zainol NR. Exploring the mass adoption potential of wearable fitness devices in Malaysia. Digit Health 2023; 920552076231180728
[http://dx.doi.org/10.1177/20552076231180728] [PMID: 37325073]

[26]   Dunning T, Duggan N, Savage S, Martin P. Diabetes and end of life: ethical and methodological issues in gathering evidence to guide care. Scand J Caring Sci 2013; 27(1): 203-11.
[http://dx.doi.org/10.1111/j.1471-6712.2012.01016.x] [PMID: 22616998]

[27]   O' Sullivan L, Feeney L, Crowley RK, Sukumar P, McAuliffe E, Doran P. An evaluation of the process of informed consent: views from research participants and staff. Trials 2021; 22(1): 544.
[http://dx.doi.org/10.1186/s13063-021-05493-1] [PMID: 34407858]

[28]   Pietrzykowski T, Smilowska K. The reality of informed consent: empirical studies on patient comprehension—systematic review. Trials 2021; 22(1): 57.
[http://dx.doi.org/10.1186/s13063-020-04969-w] [PMID: 33446265]

[29]   Corrigan O. Empty ethics: the problem with informed consent. Sociol Health Illn 2003; 25(7): 768-92.
[http://dx.doi.org/10.1046/j.1467-9566.2003.00369.x] [PMID: 19780205]

[30]   Manti S, Licari A. How to obtain informed consent for research. Breathe (Sheff) 2018; 14(2): 145-52.
[http://dx.doi.org/10.1183/20734735.001918] [PMID: 29875834]

[31]   Durand MA, Moulton B, Cockle E, Mann M, Elwyn G. Can shared decision-making reduce medical malpractice litigation? A systematic review. BMC Health Serv Res 2015; 15(1): 167.
[http://dx.doi.org/10.1186/s12913-015-0823-2] [PMID: 25927953]

[32]   Mallardi V. The origin of informed consent. Acta Otorhinolaryngol Ital organo Uff della Soc Ital di Otorinolaringol e Chir cervico-facciale; 25.

[33]   Neff MJ. Informed consent: What is it? Who can give it? How do we improve it? In: Respiratory Care. 2008.

[34]   Agozzino E, Borrelli S, Cancellieri M, Carfora FM, Di Lorenzo T, Attena F. Does written informed consent adequately inform surgical patients? A cross sectional study. BMC Med Ethics 2019; 20(1): 1.
[http://dx.doi.org/10.1186/s12910-018-0340-z] [PMID: 30616673]

[35]   Pope JE, Tingey DP, Arnold JMO, *et al.* Are subjects satisfied with the informed consent process? A survey of research participants. J Rheumatol; 30.

[36]   Verheggen FWSM, Jonkers R, Kok G. Patients' perceptions on informed consent and the quality of information disclosure in clinical trials. Patient Educ Couns 1996; 29(2): 137-53.
[http://dx.doi.org/10.1016/0738-3991(96)00859-2] [PMID: 9006231]

[37]   Grady C. Enduring and emerging challenges of informed consent. N Engl J Med 2015; 372(9): 855-62.
[http://dx.doi.org/10.1056/NEJMra1411250] [PMID: 25714163]

[38]   Miotto R, Li L, Kidd BA, Dudley JT. Deep patient: An unsupervised representation to predict the future of patients from the electronic health records. Sci Rep 2016; 6(1): 26094.
[http://dx.doi.org/10.1038/srep26094] [PMID: 27185194]

[39]   Hah H, Goldin DS. How clinicians perceive artificial intelligence–assisted technologies in diagnostic decision making: Mixed methods approach. J Med Internet Res 2021; 23(12)e33540
[http://dx.doi.org/10.2196/33540] [PMID: 34924356]

[40]   Zuocheng Wen , Hua Huang . The potential for artificial intelligence in healthcare. J Commer Biotechnol 2023; 27(4)
[http://dx.doi.org/10.5912/jcb1327]

[41] Stanfill MH, Marc DT. Health information management: Implications of artificial intelligence on healthcare data and information management. Yearb Med Inform 2019; 28(1): 056-64.
[http://dx.doi.org/10.1055/s-0039-1677913] [PMID: 31419816]

[42] Penteado BE, Fornazin M, Castro L, Rachid R. The regulation of artificial intelligence in healthcare: An exploratory study. In: Proceedings of the Association for Computing Machinery; 2023. New York (NY): ACM.
[http://dx.doi.org/10.1145/3510606.3551898]

[43] Borna S, Maniaci MJ, Haider CR, *et al.* Artificial intelligence models in health information exchange: A systematic review of clinical implications. Healthcare (Basel) 2023; 11(18): 2584.
[http://dx.doi.org/10.3390/healthcare11182584] [PMID: 37761781]

[44] Bellucci N. Disruptive innovation and technological influences on healthcare. J Radiol Nurs 2022; 41(2): 98-101.
[http://dx.doi.org/10.1016/j.jradnu.2022.02.008]

[45] Weiskopf NG, Weng C. Methods and dimensions of electronic health record data quality assessment: enabling reuse for clinical research. J Am Med Inform Assoc 2013; 20(1): 144-51.
[http://dx.doi.org/10.1136/amiajnl-2011-000681] [PMID: 22733976]

[46] Wang X, Sontag D, Wang F. Unsupervised learning of disease progression models. Proceedings of the ACM SIGKDD International Conference on Knowledge Discovery and Data Mining.
[http://dx.doi.org/10.1145/2623330.2623754]

[47] Jordan MI, Mitchell TM. Machine learning: Trends, perspectives, and prospects. Science 2015; 349(6245): 255-60.
[http://dx.doi.org/10.1126/science.aaa8415] [PMID: 26185243]

[48] Jensen PB, Jensen LJ, Brunak S. Mining electronic health records: towards better research applications and clinical care. Nat Rev Genet 2012; 13(6): 395-405.
[http://dx.doi.org/10.1038/nrg3208] [PMID: 22549152]

[49] Bellazzi R, Zupan B. Predictive data mining in clinical medicine: Current issues and guidelines. Int J Med Inform 2008; 77(2): 81-97.
[http://dx.doi.org/10.1016/j.ijmedinf.2006.11.006] [PMID: 17188928]

[50] Wang S, Šuster S, Baldwin T, Verspoor K. Predicting publication of clinical trials using structured and unstructured data: Model development and validation study. J Med Internet Res 2022; 24(12)e38859
[http://dx.doi.org/10.2196/38859] [PMID: 36563029]

[51] Blümle A, Huwiler K, Witschi M, Huwiler K, Witschi M, Egger M. Publication and non-publication of clinical trials: longitudinal study of applications submitted to a research ethics committee. Swiss Med Wkly 2008; 138(1314): 197-203.
[http://dx.doi.org/10.4414/smw.2008.12027] [PMID: 18389392]

[52] Dickersin K, Rennie D. The evolution of trial registries and their use to assess the clinical trial enterprise. JAMA 2012; 307(17): 1861-4.
[http://dx.doi.org/10.1001/jama.2012.4230] [PMID: 22550202]

[53] Mtshali S, Jacobs BA. On the validation of a fractional order model for pharmacokinetics using clinical data. Fractal Fract 2023; 7(1): 84.
[http://dx.doi.org/10.3390/fractalfract7010084]

[54] Collin CB, Gebhardt T, Golebiewski M, *et al.* Computational models for clinical applications in personalized medicine—guidelines and recommendations for data integration and model validation. J Pers Med 2022; 12(2): 166.
[http://dx.doi.org/10.3390/jpm12020166] [PMID: 35207655]

[55] Pollock RF, Norrbacka K, Boye KS, Osumili B, Valentine WJ. The PRIME Type 2 Diabetes Model: a novel, patient-level model for estimating long-term clinical and cost outcomes in patients with type 2 diabetes mellitus. J Med Econ 2022; 25(1): 393-402.

[http://dx.doi.org/10.1080/13696998.2022.2035132] [PMID: 35105267]

[56]   McEwan P, Foos V, Palmer JL, Lamotte M, Lloyd A, Grant D. Validation of the IMS CORE diabetes model. Value Health 2014; 17(6): 714-24.
[http://dx.doi.org/10.1016/j.jval.2014.07.007] [PMID: 25236995]

[57]   Palmera AJ, Rozea S, Valentinea WJ, *et al.* Validation of the CORE Diabetes Model against epidemiological and clinical studies. Curr Med Res Opin 2004; 20(sup1) (Suppl. 1): S27-40.
[http://dx.doi.org/10.1185/030079904X2006] [PMID: 15324514]

[58]   Palmer AJ, Roze S, Valentine WJ, *et al.* The CORE Diabetes Model: Projecting long-term clinical outcomes, costs and cost-effectiveness of interventions in diabetes mellitus (types 1 and 2) to support clinical and reimbursement decision-making. Curr Med Res Opin 2004; 20(sup1) (Suppl. 1): S5-S26.
[http://dx.doi.org/10.1185/030079904X1980] [PMID: 15324513]

[59]   Roick J, Ringeisen T. Self-efficacy, test anxiety, and academic success: A longitudinal validation. Int J Educ Res 2017; 83: 84-93.
[http://dx.doi.org/10.1016/j.ijer.2016.12.006]

[60]   Yates LA, Aandahl Z, Richards SA, Brook BW. Cross validation for model selection: A review with examples from ecology. Ecol Monogr 2023; 93(1)e1557
[http://dx.doi.org/10.1002/ecm.1557]

[61]   Arlot S, Celisse A. A survey of cross-validation procedures for model selection. Stat Surv 2010; 4(none)
[http://dx.doi.org/10.1214/09-SS054]

[62]   Seraj A, Mohammadi-Khanaposhtani M, Daneshfar R, *et al.* Cross-validation.Handbook of HydroInformatics. Classic Soft-Computing Techniques 2022; Vol. I: pp. 89-105.

[63]   Ramspek CL, Jager KJ, Dekker FW, Zoccali C, van Diepen M. External validation of prognostic models: what, why, how, when and where? Clin Kidney J 2021; 14(1): 49-58.
[http://dx.doi.org/10.1093/ckj/sfaa188] [PMID: 33564405]

[64]   Gramatica P. Principles of QSAR models validation: internal and external. QSAR Comb Sci 2007; 26(5): 694-701.
[http://dx.doi.org/10.1002/qsar.200610151]

[65]   Steyerberg EW, Harrell FE Jr, Borsboom GJJM, Eijkemans MJC, Vergouwe Y, Habbema JDF. Internal validation of predictive models. J Clin Epidemiol 2001; 54(8): 774-81.
[http://dx.doi.org/10.1016/S0895-4356(01)00341-9] [PMID: 11470385]

[66]   Dhafari TB, Pate A, Azadbakht N, *et al.* A scoping review finds a growing trend in studies validating multimorbidity patterns and identifies five broad types of validation methods. J Clin Epidemiol 2024; 165111214
[http://dx.doi.org/10.1016/j.jclinepi.2023.11.004] [PMID: 37952700]

[67]   Mudaranthakam DP, Phadnis MA, Krebill R, *et al.* Improving the efficiency of clinical trials by standardizing processes for Investigator Initiated Trials. Contemp Clin Trials Commun 2020; 18100579
[http://dx.doi.org/10.1016/j.conctc.2020.100579] [PMID: 32510004]

[68]   Na R, Bae JB, Jung SH, Kim KW. Clinical data interchange standards in clinical trials on alzheimer's disease. Psychiatry Investig 2022; 19(10): 814-23.
[http://dx.doi.org/10.30773/pi.2022.0149] [PMID: 36327961]

[69]   Sessler DI, Imrey PB. Clinical research methodology 2: Observational clinical research. Anesth Analg 2015; 121(4): 1043-51.
[http://dx.doi.org/10.1213/ANE.0000000000000861] [PMID: 26378704]

[70]   Kiani AK, Naureen Z, Pheby D, *et al.* Methodology for clinical research. Journal of preventive medicine and hygiene; 63. Epub ahead of print2022.
[http://dx.doi.org/10.15167/2421-4248/jpmh2022.63.2S3.2769]

[71]   Wu T, Bian Z, Li Y, *et al.* Promoting standardization of clinical trial data management in China. Chinese J Evidence-Based Med 2018; 18
[http://dx.doi.org/10.7507/1672-2531.201804096]

[72]   Chander NG. Standardization of clinical trials. J Indian Prosthodont Soc 2017; 17(1): 1-2.
[http://dx.doi.org/10.4103/0972-4052.197942] [PMID: 28216837]

[73]   Tsao MS, Carbone M, Galateau-Salle F, *et al.* Pathologic considerations and standardization in mesothelioma cinical trials. J Thorac Oncol 2019; 14(10): 1704-17.
[http://dx.doi.org/10.1016/j.jtho.2019.06.020] [PMID: 31260832]

[74]   Ghersi D. and AL. International standards for clinical trial registries. World Health Organization (WHO).

[75]   Carvalho ECA, Jayanti MK, Batilana AP, *et al.* Standardizing clinical trials workflow representation in UML for international site comparison. PLoS One 2010; 5(11)e13893
[http://dx.doi.org/10.1371/journal.pone.0013893] [PMID: 21085484]

[76]   Simalatsar A. Synthetic biomedical data generation in support of *in silico* clinical trials. Front Big Data 2023; 61085571
[http://dx.doi.org/10.3389/fdata.2023.1085571] [PMID: 37655113]

[77]   Blind E, Janssen H, Dunder K, de Graeff PA. The European Medicines Agency's approval of new medicines for type 2 diabetes. Diabetes Obes Metab 2018; 20(9): 2059-63.
[http://dx.doi.org/10.1111/dom.13349] [PMID: 29740935]

[78]   Heinemann L, Khatami H, McKinnon R, Home P. An overview of current regulatory requirements for approval of biosimilar insulins. Diabetes Technol Ther 2015; 17(7): 510-26.
[http://dx.doi.org/10.1089/dia.2014.0362] [PMID: 25789689]

[79]   Karpen SR, Dunne JL, Frohnert BI, *et al.* Consortium-based approach to receiving an EMA qualification opinion on the use of islet autoantibodies as enrichment biomarkers in type 1 diabetes clinical studies. Diabetologia 2023; 66(3): 415-24.
[http://dx.doi.org/10.1007/s00125-022-05751-0] [PMID: 35867129]

[80]   European Medicines Agency (EMA). Guideline on clinical investigation of medicinal products in the treatment or prevention of Diabetes Mellitus. Eur Med Agency; 44.

[81]   Morris LS, Schulz RM. Patient compliance-an overview. J Clin Pharm Ther 1992; 17(5): 283-95.
[http://dx.doi.org/10.1111/j.1365-2710.1992.tb01306.x] [PMID: 1464632]

CHAPTER 7

Future Scope and Innovations

Abstract: *In silico* modeling has become a ground-breaking technique in diabetes research in recent years, offering new methods for simulating, forecasting, and improving diabetic treatments. There is an urgent and unrelenting demand for more individualized, effective, and timely management options given the rise in diabetes incidence worldwide. This chapter will explore the potential of *in silico* modeling for diabetes in the future, outlining all of its most recent developments, potential innovations, and modeling pathways for collaboration with bioinformatics and Artificial Intelligence (AI). It explores the potential implications of these developments for the development of virtual clinical trials, insights into diabetes medication management, and ways to overcome the barrier of validating and integrating these models in a clinical context. We also explore the possibilities of *in silico* modeling for better regimen strategy optimization and the operation of this coupled mechanistic-phenomenological model with AI-bioinformatics for improved prediction and personalization. The chapter focuses on how these cutting-edge technologies can improve patient outcomes, clinical trial time and cost, and customized treatment. It covers a difficult spectrum, from developing and promoting regulatory settings to addressing the reproducibility of these models.

The future of diabetes care appears increasingly bright with the help of science-driven advancements in bioengineering and technology-driven drivers like AI-backed predictive analytics, multi-omics data, and virtual trial simulations.

Keywords: Artificial intelligence, Bioinformatics, Diabetes, *In silico*, Personalized treatment, Technological advancements.

INTRODUCTION

The increase in the rate of diabetes globally has catalyzed a need for personalized, effective, and timely management strategies that aid in improving outcomes. While treatment paradigms are critical, they have proven to be inadequate in managing the complexity that accompanies diabetes and its myriad of associated complications. Thankfully, the rapid developments in computational technologies, and more specifically in *in silico* modeling, have provided a disruptive approach to diabetes research by creating new avenues to model, forecast, and strategize treatments.

Darshna M. Joshi, Hardik Bhatt & Himanshu K. Patel

Novel advanced algorithms and computational frameworks facilitate the construction of virtual models of diabetic processes through *in silico* modeling. They allow for the testing of innovative pathways to treatment, simulation of clinical scenarios, and forecasting of patient-specific responses. Coupling bioinformatics and AI improves the capacity of these models to analyze more complex biological datasets. This blend of technologies has the potential to change the understanding and management of diabetes on an individual and population level.

This chapter focuses on the current trends in diabetes research that are being facilitated through *in silico* modeling, such as recent developments, scope for further innovations, and collaboration with AI and bioinformatics. In this context, we try to understand how these technologies are changing the landscape of treating diabetes diseases, from improving regimen optimization to performing virtual clinical trials. Furthermore, we cover what is still lacking, which includes model validation, regulatory hurdles, and clinical acceptance, keeping in mind how these technologies stand to redefine the value proposition in diabetes care delivery and diagnostics.

In particular, the trifecta of *in silico* modeling, AI, and bioinformatics offers tremendous promise for diabetes care. This chapter describes how these technologies can be used to improve the design of clinical trials, shorten the time needed to develop new drugs, and, most importantly, provide more effective treatment plans for diabetes patients all around the globe.

EMERGING TRENDS IN *IN SILICO* MODELING FOR DIABETES THERAPIES

A computer-based technology called "*in silico* modeling" makes it possible to use bioinformatics to analyze intricate disease mechanisms. It is possible to model drug-receptor interactions. The primary benefit of modeling is its cost-effectiveness and ability to reduce the need for expensive and time-consuming *in vitro* or *in vivo* procedures. It enables the examination of both physical and chemical properties and reduces the need for using animals in experiments [1 - 7]. Emerging trends in *in silico* modeling for diabetes therapies are shown in Table **1** [1 - 7].

Table 1. Emerging trends in *in silico* modeling [1–7]

Emerging Trend	Description	Impact	Example
Integration of AI and ML	The application of Artificial Intelligence (AI) and Machine Learning (ML) for analyzing extensive datasets and forecasting responses to therapy.	Personalized treatment, discovering drug targets, and optimizing doses by predicting how individuals will respond to therapies.	In order to manage Type 2 diabetes, AI models are being created to forecast how people will react to SGLT2 inhibitors or GLP-1 receptor agonists.
Multi-Scale Modeling	Combining data at different biological levels (*e.g.*, genomic, transcriptomic, proteomic) to simulate interactions in diabetes.	Provides more accurate models of diabetes progression and therapeutic effects across different biological scales (cellular, organ, systemic).	Multi-scale models simulating insulin resistance and its effect on metabolism and inflammation.
Personalized Medicine & Precision Therapeutics	Tailoring therapies to individuals based on genetic, environmental, and lifestyle factors.	Models predict individual responses to therapies, improving outcomes by minimizing trial and error and side effects.	Genomic-based models predicting insulin therapy effectiveness based on genetic variation.
Simulation of Disease Progression & Treatment Outcomes	Simulating long-term effects of therapies on diabetes progression and complications.	Enables accurate prediction of long-term outcomes like kidney disease, retinopathy, and cardiovascular risk.	Simulations of insulin therapy's impact on diabetic kidney disease or neuropathy progression.
Virtual Clinical Trials & Drug Repurposing	Use of *in silico* models to conduct virtual clinical trials and repurpose existing drugs for diabetes therapy.	Accelerates drug development and reduces cost by simulating the effects of drugs in virtual populations before clinical testing.	Metformin being repurposed for other conditions using *in silico* simulations, such as cancer or neurodegenerative diseases.
Integration of Real-World Data (RWD) & Digital Health	Incorporating real-time data from wearables, EHRs, and Continuous Glucose Monitors (CGMs) into models for dynamic simulation.	Enhances model accuracy by using real-world, real-time data to improve predictive power and help tailor treatments to current patient conditions.	Use of CGM data to simulate and optimize insulin therapy for Type 1 diabetes or Type 2 diabetes.
Advanced Computational Methods & Quantum Computing	Application of quantum computing and High-performance Computing (HPC) for complex simulations of disease mechanisms and drug interactions.	Enables the simulation of more complex biological systems, speeding up the drug discovery process and improving precision in diabetes therapy development.	Use of quantum algorithms to predict protein-ligand interactions for developing novel insulin analogs.

Personalized treatments have improved as a result of the incorporation of AI and ML techniques into model creation. Additionally, data from different biological layers are combined using multiscale modeling. Models based on genetic and other individual variables can be used to forecast personalized treatment. It is possible to mimic long-term illness prognosis and drug effects. Virtual trials increase the effectiveness of drug development. Additionally, the model can incorporate real-world data to enable more precise and accurate drug discovery [8 - 21].

POTENTIAL IMPACTS AND INNOVATIONS IN DIABETES MANAGEMENT

Novel approaches, like *in silico* modeling, are redefining diabetes management as the world grows more technologically advanced. When paired with other advances, emerging technologies hold the potential to improve diabetes patients' quality of life, treatment efficacy, and outcomes. An outline of the main effects and developments in diabetes care brought about by advances in data science, technology, and biomedical research is presented. Table **2** [22] shows the impact and description of personalized and precision medicine with examples [22]. Table **3** [23] shows the impact on enhanced disease progression [23]. Drug discovery and repurposing are explained in Table **4** [24].

Table 2. Personalized and precision medicine [22].

Impact	Description	Innovation Example
Tailored Therapies	*In silico* models assist in customizing treatments for individual patients by examining their genetic information, lifestyle choices, and medical history.	Genomic-based models can forecast how individuals will respond to various diabetes medications, including insulin and GLP-1 receptor agonists, by considering their genetic predispositions.
Better Patient Outcomes	Personalized treatment plans minimize the trial-and-error process, resulting in quicker and more effective management of blood sugar levels.	Machine learning algorithms can enhance drug dosing and forecast which treatments will yield the most beneficial long-term outcomes for individual patients.

Table 3. Enhanced disease progression monitoring [23].

Impact	Description	Innovation Example
Predictive Analytics	*In silico* models can mimic disease progression and assess the effects of different interventions over time, offering real-time insights.	Simulation tools can forecast the impact of various diabetes treatments on long-term outcomes, including the onset of diabetic nephropathy or retinopathy.

(Table 3) cont.....

Impact	Description	Innovation Example
Early Detection of Complications	Through real-time modeling, clinicians can detect early signs of complications and adjust treatments to prevent them.	By using real-time modeling, healthcare providers can identify early signs of complications and modify treatments to avert them.

Table 4. Drug discovery and repurposing [24].

Impact	Description	Innovation Example
Faster Drug Development	Virtual screening and *in silico* models speed up the process of discovering new drug candidates by simulating how they interact with biological targets.	AI-driven drug discovery is uncovering potential new compounds for diabetes treatment, significantly cutting down the time and cost associated with bringing new therapies to market.
Drug Repurposing	Existing medications can be evaluated for their effectiveness in addressing complications related to diabetes, offering quick treatment alternatives.	*In silico* modeling has revealed promising repurposed drugs, such as metformin, that could be effective in treating not only diabetes but also cancer and neurodegenerative diseases.

Real-time continuous monitoring is explained in Table **5** [25], while the impact of AI and ML in clinical decision support is shown in Table **6** [26]. Description regarding patient engagement is shown in Table **7** [27], and Table **8** [9] shows the impact of virtual trials. Regulatory advancements are shown in Table **9** [27], and global healthcare accessibility is shown in Table **10** [7].

Table 5. Real-time and continuous monitoring [25].

Impact	Description	Innovation Example
24/7 Monitoring	The integration of wearable devices like Continuous Glucose Monitors (CGMs) and smart insulin pens allows for ongoing tracking of glucose levels and insulin usage.	Continuous Glucose Monitoring (CGM) systems offer real-time information that helps both patients and healthcare providers make informed decisions about treatment adjustments.
Dynamic Treatment Adjustment	Real-time data from wearables and sensors enables automatic therapy adjustments, reducing the chances of hypoglycemia or hyperglycemia.	Closed-loop insulin systems automatically adjust insulin delivery using real-time glucose readings, allowing for tighter glucose control with minimal intervention.

Table 6. AI and Machine Learning in Clinical Decision Support [26].

Impact	Description	Innovation Example
Enhanced Decision-Making	AI models offer clinicians valuable insights based on data to aid in complex decision-making, including the best therapy choices and appropriate dosages.	Clinical Decision Support Systems (CDSS) that utilize AI provide tailored therapy suggestions based on individual patient data, enhancing outcomes and minimizing errors.
Prediction of Treatment Response	AI and machine learning models forecast how patients will react to various treatments, enhancing the accuracy of interventions.	Predictive models utilize patient data to anticipate responses to insulin therapy, aiding in the optimization of treatment prior to the onset of complications.

Table 7. Improved patient engagement and education [27].

Impact	Description	Innovation Example
Empowered Patients	Mobile apps and platforms powered by *in silico* models enable patients to take an active role in monitoring and managing their health in partnership with healthcare providers.	Diabetes management apps that combine data from wearables, food diaries, and exercise habits to provide patients with insights into their health and the effectiveness of their treatment.
Behavioural Insights	Data-driven tools provide valuable insights into patient behavior, enabling healthcare providers to develop personalized education plans that enhance adherence.	Smartphone apps that offer real-time feedback on diet, exercise, and medication adherence can enhance patient engagement and support self-management.

Table 8. Virtual clinical trials [9].

Impact	Description	Innovation Example
Cost-Effective Trials	Virtual trials, utilizing *in silico* modeling, create simulations of clinical trials within virtual populations, which help to cut down on both costs and time in the drug development process.	Virtual clinical trials for diabetes medications utilize simulation software to forecast the effectiveness and safety of these drugs across various patient groups.
Faster Patient Recruitment	*In silico* models mimic how patients respond to treatments, aiding in the identification of the best candidates for real-world trials, which in turn accelerates recruitment.	The use of simulation-based recruitment in virtual trials for drugs aimed at treating Type 1 or Type 2 diabetes, utilizing genetic and clinical data.

Table 9. Regulatory advancements and digital health integration [27].

Impact	Description	Innovation Example
Regulatory Flexibility	Recent advancements *in silico* modeling and digital health tools are promoting more flexible and adaptive regulatory pathways for products related to diabetes.	The FDA has approved digital therapeutics, such as mobile apps and software-based interventions, for managing diabetes, which has shortened the time it takes to bring new solutions to market.
Real-Time Regulatory Monitoring	Continuous patient monitoring through wearables and sensors can provide real-time data for regulatory bodies to track the safety and efficacy of diabetes therapies.	Real-time data collection and analysis using Continuous Glucose Monitors (CGMs) and smart insulin pumps provide ongoing feedback to regulatory bodies regarding the safety of diabetes treatments.

Table 10. Global healthcare accessibility [7].

Impact	Description	Innovation Example
Broadening Access to Care	*In silico* models facilitate the creation of affordable therapies, while digital health solutions can extend diabetes care to populations that are often overlooked.	Telemedicine platforms that incorporate *in silico* diabetes management tools enable remote monitoring and care, making it easier for individuals in rural or underserved areas to manage their diabetes.
Affordable and Scalable Solutions	Digital tools and virtual trials help lower costs, enabling more affordable treatments and increasing the scalability of interventions for global populations.	AI-driven mobile platforms offer cost-effective diabetes management solutions in low-resource environments, with the potential to assist millions of underserved individuals around the globe.

Real-time monitoring, AI-powered clinical decision assistance, virtual trials, tailored treatment, and enhanced drug development are just a few of the many possible advances and effects in diabetes care. Diabetes management is becoming more effective, accurate, and scalable thanks to *in silico* modeling and the incorporation of cutting-edge technologies like Artificial Intelligence (AI), machine learning, and wearable technology. By enhancing patient outcomes, increasing accessibility, and reducing healthcare costs, these innovations will revolutionize diabetes care and eventually make diabetes management more patient-centred, data-driven, and individualized globally [28 - 32].

VIRTUAL TRIALS IN DIABETES MANAGEMENT

Virtual Clinical Trials (VCTs) are a novel approach that uses data modeling, digital tools, and remote monitoring technologies to collect data and duplicate clinical trials in real-world environments without the need for conventional in-person visits. Because it can speed up medication development, reduce expenses, and increase patient access to clinical trials—especially for chronic illnesses like diabetes—this method is gaining traction in diabetes research. For remote data collection and analysis, VCTs rely heavily on wearable technology, digital health platforms, and *in silico* modeling [33 - 39]. Various factors in virtual trials for diabetes management are shown in Table **11**[9].

Table 11. Virtual trials components [9].

Component	Description	Benefits
Patient Recruitment	Virtual trials utilize data-driven algorithms to find and enroll suitable participants based on particular criteria, such as genetic, demographic, and clinical information. Patients have the option to participate remotely through telemedicine or online platforms.	Accelerated recruitment using focused, data-informed strategies. - Expanded participant pool, encompassing both global and underserved communities. - Involvement of patients who may lack access to conventional trials.
Remote Monitoring Devices	Wearable technologies like Continuous Glucose Monitors (CGMs), smart insulin pumps, and mobile health apps are designed to continuously track vital signs, glucose levels, and other important parameters right from patients' homes.	Continuous, real-time data collection. - Decreased necessity for in-person visits. - Enhanced accuracy in real-time insights regarding treatment effects and adverse events.
Digital Health Platforms	Mobile apps and online platforms play a crucial role in enhancing patient engagement, tracking therapy adherence, and offering immediate feedback to both patients and healthcare providers. Additionally, these platforms have the capability to gather qualitative data.	Patient engagement is enhanced through intuitive interfaces. - Provides real-time feedback and guidance. - Boosts adherence by sending reminders and facilitating direct communication with healthcare teams.
***In Silico* Modeling and Simulation**	Virtual trials can utilize *in silico* models to mimic how patients respond to treatments, forecast outcomes, and enhance the design of clinical trials. These computational models replicate real-world situations, allowing for testing on virtual populations.	- Cut costs by simulating drug effects prior to physical trials. - Gained predictive insights for clinical trial results. - Modeled rare patient populations or complex conditions that are challenging to recruit in traditional trials.
Data Integration and Analysis	In virtual trials, data collected from various sources like Continuous Glucose Monitors (CGMs), smart devices, and surveys are integrated into a central database. This enables real-time analysis using Artificial Intelligence (AI) and Machine Learning (ML).	- Automated data analysis allows for quicker decision-making. - Tailored treatment suggestions based on up-to-date patient information. - Effective and precise outcome assessment through ongoing monitoring.

Virtual clinical trials are changing the way diabetes therapies are researched, developed, and tested. By using remote monitoring tools, digital health platforms, and *in silico* models, these trials provide significant benefits such as cost savings, faster timelines, and broader patient access. As virtual trials continue to develop, they have the potential to enhance the efficiency and inclusivity of diabetes research, making patient-centred care more personalized and effective. However, it is crucial to pay close attention to data security and regulatory compliance, ensuring that all populations can participate in this innovative approach to clinical testing.

ADDRESSING CHALLENGES AND COMPLEXITIES IN THE VALIDATION OF *IN SILICO* MODELS FOR DIABETES

In silico models are now essential for diabetes research, medication development, and therapy plan customization. These computer programs estimate the course of diseases, model biological systems, and improve treatment plans. However, the complexity of diabetes, the range of patient demographics, and the need for precise, dependable, and therapeutically meaningful data make validating *in silico* models extremely difficult. For these models to be accepted in clinical practice, their reliability and reproducibility must be guaranteed. The challenge associated with the models and the solution to the same is provided in Table **12** [40]. Lack of sufficient data also imposes a major challenge, which is covered in Table **13** [41]. Validation against clinical outcomes is the most important for each computational model. The challenge with the same is explained in Table **14** [40]. Regulatory and ethical considerations are considered during validation, which is shown in Table **15** [42]. Selection of modeling methodologies is one of the important tasks that faces many challenges. The solution is discussed in Table **16** [43]. Once the model is created, the reproducibility and robustness of the model are important. The same is covered in Table **17** [44].

Table 12. Model accuracy and predictive power [40].

Challenge	Description	Solution
Biological Complexity	Diabetes is a multifactorial disease involving complex interactions between genetics, lifestyle, environment, and metabolic pathways. Modeling these intricate systems accurately is difficult.	Multiscale modeling: Integrating genomic, proteomic, transcriptomic, and phenotypic data to simulate the complex biology of diabetes. Use of AI/ML to improve predictive accuracy by analyzing large datasets and identifying subtle patterns.
Data Integration	Diabetes models often require the integration of data from multiple sources (*e.g.*, clinical trials, real-world data, laboratory experiments, electronic health records), which can be inconsistent or incomplete.	Data harmonization: Standardize data formats and ensure consistency across different datasets. Use of advanced machine learning algorithms to handle missing or noisy data effectively.

(Table 12) cont.....

Challenge	Description	Solution
Model Overfitting	Overfitting occurs when a model is too closely aligned with training data, failing to generalize well to new, unseen patient data.	Cross-validation techniques to ensure that models are generalized and robust. - Use of external validation cohorts from diverse populations to test model performance.

Table 13. Lack of sufficient and high-quality data [41].

Challenge	Description	Solution
Limited Real-World Data (RWD)	While clinical trial data is highly controlled, real-world data is often messy, less structured, and inconsistent. This makes it challenging to build predictive models that apply to everyday patient populations.	Incorporate real-world evidence from patient registries, healthcare systems, and wearable devices to enhance model accuracy. - Develop data-sharing frameworks to pool data across institutions.
Data Scarcity for Rare Cases	There is a lack of data for rare forms of diabetes (*e.g.*, neonatal diabetes, maturity-onset diabetes of the young), which makes it difficult to validate models for these conditions.	Use synthetic data generation methods to simulate rare disease cases. - Implement transfer learning from well-studied subtypes of diabetes to rarer forms.
Longitudinal Data Requirements	Diabetes requires long-term data to understand progression and treatment responses, but longitudinal datasets are often scarce or incomplete.	Collaborate with long-term cohorts, such as Diabetes Prevention Programs (DPP) and Framingham Heart Study, to access large-scale longitudinal data. - Leverage retrospective studies to supplement long-term data collection.

Table 14. Validation against clinical outcomes [40].

Challenge	Description	Solution
Clinical Endpoint Measurement	*In silico* models often rely on surrogate markers (*e.g.*, HbA1c levels, insulin sensitivity) instead of hard clinical outcomes (*e.g.*, cardiovascular events, kidney failure, mortality), which can make validation difficult.	- Incorporate long-term clinical outcomes in model validation to ensure real-world relevance. - Use surrogate endpoints in conjunction with clinical trials to validate model predictions (*e.g.*, predicting long-term cardiovascular risk).
External Validation	Models that work well in one dataset or clinical cohort may not perform as well when applied to other populations, especially in diverse patient groups with different genetic, environmental, or lifestyle factors.	- Test models on external cohorts with diverse demographics and disease subtypes to ensure broader applicability. - Use global health data and diverse clinical trial populations to assess model generalizability.

(Table 14) cont.....

Challenge	Description	Solution
Clinical Integration	Even if a model is validated, integrating it into clinical workflows to influence decision-making requires additional validation of its usability and clinical utility.	- Collaborate with clinicians and healthcare providers to conduct real-world validation of model-based recommendations. - Conduct user experience studies to ensure model outputs are actionable and useful in clinical practice.

Table 15. Regulatory and ethical considerations [42].

Challenge	Description	Solution
Regulatory Approval	Regulatory agencies (*e.g.*, FDA, EMA) require evidence that *in silico* models are validated and reliable before they can be used for clinical decision-making or as part of regulatory submissions.	- Collaborate with regulatory bodies early in the development process to establish guidelines for *in silico* validation. - Perform prospective studies and publish results in peer-reviewed journals to gain acceptance.
Ethical Considerations	Ensuring that *in silico* models are transparent, accountable, and free from bias is crucial, especially when they are used to influence treatment decisions or predict outcomes.	- Ensure model transparency through open-source frameworks and detailed model documentation. - Regularly audit models for bias and fairness by examining model performance across diverse demographic groups.

Table 16. Complexities in standardizing modeling methodologies [43].

Challenge	Description	Solution
Lack of Standard Protocols	The heterogeneity of *in silico* modeling approaches, including different algorithms, simulation techniques, and data inputs, makes it difficult to achieve a standardized methodology.	- Develop best practices and standardized protocols for model development and validation (*e.g.*, model verification and validation procedures). - Use open-source platforms and interoperable tools to promote consistency across models.
Model Complexity *vs.* Usability	More complex models can provide greater predictive power but may lack clinical usability due to their difficulty in interpreting or implementing in a clinical setting.	- Focus on creating clinically interpretable models that balance complexity with practicality in decision-making. - Engage with clinicians throughout the model development process to ensure that outputs are actionable.
Model Interpretability	Complex models, especially those using AI and machine learning, can act as "black boxes," making it difficult for clinicians to understand the reasoning behind predictions or recommendations.	- Incorporate Explainable AI (XAI) techniques into models, providing clinicians with interpretability and transparency on how decisions are made. - Use visualizations and user-friendly interfaces to make model outputs more accessible.

Table 17. Model reproducibility and robustness [44].

Challenge	Description	Solution
Reproducibility Across Cohorts	Ensuring that *in silico* models can be replicated across different datasets, institutions, or time periods is a significant challenge.	- Conduct sensitivity analysis to test model robustness under various conditions. - Use cross-site validation and multi-institution collaborations to test models across different cohorts and datasets.
Environmental Variability	Diabetes models may perform well under controlled conditions but fail when exposed to environmental variability (*e.g.*, changes in population demographics or healthcare settings).	- Incorporate heterogeneous data from different environments, patient populations, and regions to improve model generalizability. - Design models that are adaptive to evolving clinical practices and demographic shifts.

The complexity of biological systems and the need for high-quality, long-term data present significant challenges in validating *in silico* models for diabetes management. To tackle these issues, a comprehensive approach is necessary, which includes advanced data integration, collaboration with regulatory and clinical organizations, and the development of standardized validation methods. Additionally, ensuring the clinical value, reproducibility, and transparency of these models is crucial for their widespread adoption in clinical practice. Addressing these challenges can revolutionize diabetes care by enabling more personalized treatments, enhancing clinical trials, and improving patient outcomes [44 - 53].

ARTIFICIAL INTELLIGENCE AND BIOINFORMATICS IN *IN SILICO* MODELING

In silico modeling using bioinformatics and Artificial Intelligence (AI) has revolutionized diabetes research and treatment development. The modeling, prediction, and optimization of diabetes treatment strategies are made possible by AI's capacity to evaluate vast datasets and generate predictions, in conjunction with the advanced computational tools of bioinformatics. Diabetes care is becoming more precise and individualized thanks to these advancements. This section looks at the benefits and drawbacks of AI and bioinformatics in improving *in silico* models for diabetes [26, 54 - 61]. The role of AI and bioinformatics in the modeling of diabetes is shown in Table **18** [62] and Table **19**, respectively [63].

Table 18. Role of artificial intelligence in *in silico* modeling for diabetes [62].

AI Technique	Description	Application in Diabetes
Machine Learning (ML)	Machine learning algorithms allow models to learn patterns from data without being explicitly programmed. This is especially useful for handling the vast, complex datasets in diabetes care.	- Prediction of treatment outcomes: ML algorithms predict how individual patients will respond to different diabetes therapies, optimizing treatment choices. - Early detection of complications: Predicting the onset of complications like diabetic retinopathy or nephropathy using patient data.
Deep Learning (DL)	A subfield of ML that uses neural networks to model highly complex, non-linear relationships. DL is effective in extracting features from large, unstructured datasets like images, genomic data, and time-series data.	- Image analysis: DL models can analyze retina scans to detect diabetic retinopathy. - Genomic data analysis: DL models can identify genetic factors contributing to diabetes susceptibility.
Reinforcement Learning (RL)	Reinforcement learning involves training models to make decisions by interacting with an environment and receiving feedback based on the actions taken. This technique is particularly useful for dynamic and adaptive systems like diabetes therapy management.	- Personalized treatment regimens: RL can be used to develop adaptive insulin dosing strategies, adjusting doses based on real-time glucose data. - Simulation of long-term treatment strategies to optimize disease management.
Natural Language Processing (NLP)	NLP enables computers to process and understand human language. It is applied to structured and unstructured textual data, such as medical records and research publications.	- Mining Electronic Health Records (EHRs): Extracting useful insights from unstructured clinical data to predict disease progression or recommend treatment adjustments. - Clinical decision support: NLP can assist in generating evidence-based treatment recommendations from literature or medical notes.
Predictive Analytics	Predictive analytics uses statistical algorithms and machine learning techniques to analyze historical data and forecast future outcomes.	Glucose forecasting: AI-powered models predict blood glucose fluctuations and adjust insulin regimens in real time. - Predicting disease progression: Using patient data to forecast long-term outcomes such as complications from Type 1 or Type 2 diabetes.

Table 19. Role of bioinformatics in *in silico* modeling for diabetes [63].

Bioinformatics Technique	Description	Application in Diabetes
Genomics and Transcriptomics	Bioinformatics tools allow researchers to analyze large-scale genetic data (*e.g.*, whole-genome sequencing, transcriptomics) to identify genetic predispositions and biomarkers for diseases.	- Genetic susceptibility: Identifying genes associated with diabetes (*e.g.*, TCF7L2, KCNJ11) and using this information to develop genetically tailored treatment plans. - Biomarker discovery: Identifying biomarkers for early diagnosis or prognosis in diabetes patients, improving personalized care.
Proteomics	The study of the proteome, or the entire set of proteins expressed in a cell, tissue, or organism. It helps in understanding the molecular mechanisms of diabetes.	- Biomarker identification: Identifying protein markers of insulin resistance or beta-cell dysfunction. - Diabetes complications: Understanding the proteomic changes related to complications such as diabetic nephropathy or cardiovascular diseases.
Metabolomics	Metabolomics involves the study of small molecules (metabolites) within a biological system and how these metabolites are altered in diseases like diabetes.	- Metabolic profiling: Profiling metabolites in patients to predict diabetes onset, progression, or response to therapy. - Personalized nutrition: Designing diet plans based on the metabolomic profile of patients to improve diabetes management.
Systems Biology	This interdisciplinary approach uses computational models to understand complex biological systems and their interactions, providing insights into disease mechanisms.	- Pathway modeling: Using *in silico* models to simulate biological pathways involved in insulin resistance, glucose metabolism, and beta-cell function. - Multi-omics integration: Combining genomic, transcriptomic, proteomic, and metabolomic data to create a comprehensive model of diabetes.
Pharmacogenomics	Pharmacogenomics involves studying how genes affect individual responses to drugs. It enables personalized drug therapies.	- Drug response prediction: Identifying genetic variations that affect responses to diabetes medications, like metformin or GLP-1 receptor agonists. - Optimizing drug therapy: Using genetic data to select the most effective medications with the fewest side effects for each patient.

By fusing the biological insights provided by computational biology with the predictive capability of machine learning algorithms, AI and bioinformatics enhance one another. Their collaboration is especially beneficial when it comes to diabetes research and management. The synergy area is covered in Table **20** [64].The challenges and limitations associated with the use of AI and bioinformatics in *in silico* modeling for diabetes are shown in Table **21** [65, 66].

Table 20. Synergy of AI and bioinformatics in *in silico* modeling for diabetes [64].

Synergy Area	Description	Application in Diabetes
Personalized Medicine	AI models can process and analyze vast amounts of data from genomic, transcriptomic, and metabolomic sources to develop highly personalized treatment strategies for diabetes patients.	- Precision therapy: AI-based analysis of genomic and phenotypic data to recommend personalized insulin regimens, lifestyle interventions, and drug therapies. - Precision nutrition: Developing diet plans tailored to individual metabolic profiles.
Omics Data Integration	By combining data from various omics technologies (genomics, proteomics, metabolomics), AI can reveal complex biological relationships and predict disease trajectories.	- Multi-omics models: AI-driven integration of genetic, proteomic, and metabolomic data to create a unified model for predicting diabetes progression and personalized treatment strategies.
Drug Discovery and Repurposing	AI models trained on bioinformatics data can simulate drug interactions with biological targets, accelerating the identification of new drugs or repurposing existing ones for diabetes.	- AI-guided drug discovery: Using AI to analyze large-scale genomic and proteomic data to identify new drug candidates or repurpose existing drugs (*e.g.*, metformin) for additional therapeutic indications.
Biomarker Identification	AI algorithms can identify patterns within omics data to discover new biomarkers that aid in early detection, prognosis, or prediction of treatment responses.	- Early biomarkers: AI-enhanced analysis of genomic, proteomic, and metabolomic data to identify new biomarkers for early diagnosis of Type 2 diabetes or diabetes complications.
Disease Modeling	*In silico* models powered by AI can simulate complex disease mechanisms based on bioinformatics data, helping researchers predict disease progression and test therapeutic interventions.	- Diabetes progression models: AI-powered *in silico* models simulate the progression of insulin resistance, beta-cell dysfunction, and other mechanisms to predict disease outcomes and optimize interventions.

Table 21. Challenges and limitations of AI and bioinformatics in *in silico* modeling for diabetes [65, 66].

Challenge	Description	Solution
Data Quality and Availability	High-quality, large-scale datasets are necessary for training AI models, but data may be limited, biased, or incomplete.	- Encourage the sharing of high-quality, annotated data from diverse populations. - Develop synthetic datasets for rare diabetes subtypes and complications.
Model Interpretability	Some AI algorithms, particularly deep learning models, can be difficult to interpret, limiting their clinical application.	- Incorporate Explainable AI (XAI) techniques to make AI models more interpretable for clinicians. - Use visual analytics to help clinicians understand model predictions.

(Table 21) cont.....

Challenge	Description	Solution
Overfitting and Generalization	AI models may perform well on training data but struggle to generalize to new or unseen patient populations.	- Use cross-validation and external validation datasets to ensure generalizability. - Regularly update models with new patient data to improve accuracy.
Integration into Clinical Workflow	Despite their potential, AI and bioinformatics models may face challenges when integrated into clinical settings	

Machine learning and bioinformatics are important enhancers of *in silico* models for diabetes by enhancing predictive power, enabling personalized treatment strategies, and improving drug discovery. Together, they provide a wide platform to understand diabetes on the molecular, cellular, and systemic levels of its occurrence. With growth in technologies, the integration of AI with bioinformatics is set to advance the domain of diabetes care well into more effective and personalized treatments. However, to achieve their fullest potential in delivering better health outcomes for patients, a few challenges regarding data quality, interpretability, and clinical integration need to be addressed [67 - 70].

CONCLUDING REMARKS

A significant change is about to occur in the realm of *in silico* modeling for diabetic treatments. Traditional treatment approaches are under pressure to offer more individualized, flexible, and accurate care as diabetes and its related disorders get more complicated. There are intriguing prospects to increase predictive accuracy and develop individualized treatment regimens by integrating bioinformatics and Artificial Intelligence (AI) into *in silico* models. Diabetes therapy testing is about to undergo a transformation thanks to new trends like virtual clinical trials, which will expedite drug discovery and reduce the need for extensive, resource-intensive trials. We must, however, address important concerns with data quality, model validation, and regulatory compliance if we are to fully realize the potential of these models. Although bioinformatics and artificial intelligence enable the creation of sophisticated models that integrate complex biological data, their successful application in clinical settings necessitates an emphasis on model interpretability, accessibility, and smooth integration with medical procedures. Furthermore, there are pressing issues that must be resolved, such as standardizing modeling methodologies and guaranteeing uniform validation across different patient groups. Despite these obstacles, *in silico* modeling has a promising future in diabetes care. With the use of accurate AI-driven models, personalized medicine has the potential to revolutionize diabetes treatment by improving patient-specific and efficacious therapies. In addition to expanding our knowledge of disease mechanisms, *in silico* modeling will help identify new therapeutic targets and advance current therapies. Collaboration between data scientists, physicians, and regulatory bodies will be essential as the area develops in order to create dependable, scalable, and therapeutically applicable models. A bright future is guaranteed by the continuous fusion of diabetes research with computational technology, which will keep opening up new possibilities in precision medicine.

CONSENT FOR PUBLICATION

We hereby give consent for publication.

DECLARATION

I utilized AI to present comprehensive information in an easy-to-understand and well-organized manner. The table's content for the paper is created using AI. It is challenging to discuss them in paragraphs.

REFERENCES

[1]   Tiwari P. Recent trends in therapeutic approaches for diabetes management: A comprehensive update. Journal of Diabetes Research 2015.
[http://dx.doi.org/10.1155/2015/340838]

[2]   Rodríguez-Rodríguez I, Campo-Valera M, Rodríguez JV, Lok Woo W. IoMT innovations in diabetes management: Predictive models using wearable data. Expert Syst Appl 2024; 238: 121994.
[http://dx.doi.org/10.1016/j.eswa.2023.121994]

[3]   Agarwal S, Griffith ML, Murphy EJ, Greenlee C, Boord J, Gabbay RA. Innovations in diabetes care for a better 'new normal' beyond COVID-19. J Clin Endocrinol Metab 2021; 106(1): e377-81.
[http://dx.doi.org/10.1210/clinem/dgaa704] [PMID: 33205818]

[4]   Mulvaney SA, Ritterband LM, Bosslet L. Mobile intervention design in diabetes: review and recommendations. Curr Diab Rep. 2011; 11: 486-493.
[http://dx.doi.org/10.1007/s11892-011-0230-y]

[5]   Zarkogianni K, Litsa E, Mitsis K, *et al.* A review of emerging technologies for the management of diabetes mellitus. IEEE Trans Biomed Eng. 2015;62(12):2735-2749.
[http://dx.doi.org/10.1109/TBME.2015.2470521]

[6]   Das L, Bhadada SK. Current advances and future avenues in endocrinology. In: Sobti R, Ganju AK, editors. Biomedical translational research. Singapore: Springer; 2022.
[http://dx.doi.org/10.1007/978-981-16-8845-4_3]

[7]   Istepanian RSH, Casiglia D, Gregory JW. Mobile health (m-Health) for diabetes management. British Journal of Healthcare Management 2017; 23(3): 102-8.
[http://dx.doi.org/10.12968/bjhc.2017.23.3.102]

[8]   Choi S, Kang CY, Lee BJ, Park JB. *In vitro-in vivo* correlation using *in silico* modeling of physiological properties, metabolites, and intestinal metabolism. Curr Drug Metab 2018; 18(11): 973-82.
[http://dx.doi.org/10.2174/1389200218666171031124347] [PMID: 29086683]

[9]   Simalatsar A. Synthetic biomedical data generation in support of *In Silico* Clinical Trials. Frontiers in Big Data 2023; 6: 1085571.

[http://dx.doi.org/10.3389/fdata.2023.1085571] [PMID: 37655113]

[10]   Haghighi O, Moradi M. *In silico* study of the structure and ligand interactions of alcohol dehydrogenase from *Cyanobacterium synechocystis sp.* PCC 6803 as a key enzyme for biofuel production. Appl Biochem Biotechnol 2020; 192(4): 1346-67.
[http://dx.doi.org/10.1007/s12010-020-03400-z] [PMID: 32767175]

[11]   Haghighi O. *In silico* study of the structure and ligand preference of pyruvate kinases from *Cyanobacterium synechocystis sp.* PCC 6803. Appl Biochem Biotechnol 2021; 193(11): 3651-71.
[http://dx.doi.org/10.1007/s12010-021-03630-9] [PMID: 34347252]

[12]   Nabati F, Moradi M, Mohabatkar H. *In silico* analyzing the molecular interactions of plant-derived inhibitors against E6AP, p53, and c-Myc binding sites of HPV type 16 E6 oncoprotein. Mol Biol Res Commun 2020; 9(2): 71-82.
[http://dx.doi.org/10.22099/mbrc.2020.36522.1483] [PMID: 32802901]

[13]   Dassau E, Palerm CC, Zisser H, Buckingham BA, Jovanovič L, Doyle FJ III. *In silico* evaluation platform for artificial pancreatic β-cell development--a dynamic simulator for closed-loop control with hardware-in-the-loop. Diabetes Technol Ther 2009; 11(3): 187-94.
[http://dx.doi.org/10.1089/dia.2008.0055] [PMID: 19191486]

[14]   Behbahani M, Moradi M, Mohabatkar H. *In silico* design of a multi-epitope peptide construct as a potential vaccine candidate for Influenza A based on neuraminidase protein. *In Silico* Pharmacol 2021; 9(1): 36.
[http://dx.doi.org/10.1007/s40203-021-00095-w] [PMID: 33987075]

[15]   Schiavon M, Man CD, Kudva YC, Basu A, Cobelli C. *In silico* optimization of basal insulin infusion rate during exercise: implication for artificial pancreas. J Diabetes Sci Technol 2013; 7(6): 1461-9.
[http://dx.doi.org/10.1177/193229681300700606] [PMID: 24351172]

[16]   de Godoi RS, Almerão MP, da Silva FR. *In silico* evaluation of the antidiabetic activity of natural compounds from Hovenia dulcis Thunberg. J Herb Med 2021; 28: 100349.
[http://dx.doi.org/10.1016/j.hermed.2020.100349]

[17]   Timo GO, Reis RSSV, Melo AF, Costa TVL, Magalhães PO, Homem-de-Mello M. Predictive power of *in silico* approach to evaluate chemicals against m. tuberculosis: A systematic review. Pharmaceuticals (Basel) 2019; 12(3): 135.
[http://dx.doi.org/10.3390/ph12030135] [PMID: 31527425]

[18]   Medeiros I, Aguiar AJFC, Fortunato WM, *et al. In silico* structure-based design of peptides or proteins as therapeutic tools for obesity or diabetes mellitus: A protocol for systematic review and meta analysis. Medicine (Baltimore) 2023; 102(15): e33514.
[http://dx.doi.org/10.1097/MD.0000000000033514] [PMID: 37058011]

[19]   Choi K, Oh TJ, Lee JC, *et al. In-silico* trials for glucose control in hospitalized patients with type 2 diabetes. J Korean Med Sci 2016; 31(2): 231-9.
[http://dx.doi.org/10.3346/jkms.2016.31.2.231] [PMID: 26839477]

[20]   Riyaphan J, Pham DC, Leong MK, Weng CF. *In silico* approaches to identify polyphenol compounds as α-glucosidase and α-amylase inhibitors against type-ii diabetes. Biomolecules 2021; 11(12): 1877.
[http://dx.doi.org/10.3390/biom11121877] [PMID: 34944521]

[21]   Campos-Náñez E, Layne JE, Zisser HC. *In silico* modeling of minimal effective insulin doses using the UVA/Padova type 1 diabetes simulator. J Diabetes Sci Technol. 2017; 12(2): 376–380.
[http://dx.doi.org/10.1177/1932296817735341]

[22]   Nielsen J. Systems biology of metabolism: A driver for developing personalized and precision medicine. Cell Metab 2017; 25(3): 572-9.
[http://dx.doi.org/10.1016/j.cmet.2017.02.002] [PMID: 28273479]

[23]   Mannino GC, Andreozzi F, Sesti G. Pharmacogenetics of type 2 diabetes mellitus, the route toward tailored medicine. Diabetes Metab Res Rev 2019; 35(3): e3109.

[http://dx.doi.org/10.1002/dmrr.3109] [PMID: 30515958]

[24]   Gangrade D, Sawant G, Mehta A. Re-thinking drug discovery: *In silico* method J Chem Pharm Res 8. Available from: www.jocpr.com

[25]   Guerrero-Arroyo L, Faulds E, Perez-Guzman MC, Davis GM, Dungan K, Pasquel FJ. Continuous glucose monitoring in the intensive care unit. J Diabetes Sci Technol 2023; 17(3): 667-78. [http://dx.doi.org/10.1177/19322968231169522] [PMID: 37081830]

[26]   Shukur BS, Yaacob NM, Doheir M. Diabetes at a glance: assessing AI strategies for early diabetes detection and intervention. Mesopotamian J Artif Intell Healthc [Internet]. 2023 Dec 10 [cited 2026 Jan 16];2023:85–9. Available from: https://doi.org/10.58496/MJAIH/2023/017

[27]   Sarani Rad F, Hendawi R, Yang X, Li J. Personalized diabetes management with digital twins: A patient-centric knowledge graph approach. J Pers Med 2024; 14(4): 359. [http://dx.doi.org/10.3390/jpm14040359] [PMID: 38672986]

[28]   Wake DJ, Gibb FW, Kar P, *et al.* ENDOCRINOLOGY IN THE TIME OF COVID-19: Remodelling diabetes services and emerging innovation. Eur J Endocrinol 2020; 183(2): G67-77. [http://dx.doi.org/10.1530/EJE-20-0377] [PMID: 32508313]

[29]   Basudev N. Shaping the future of diabetes care: innovation, people and partnerships. Pract Diabetes 2021; 38(6): 10-5. [http://dx.doi.org/10.1002/pdi.2365]

[30]   Drucker DJ. Transforming type 1 diabetes: the next wave of innovation. Diabetologia 2021; 64(5): 1059-65. [http://dx.doi.org/10.1007/s00125-021-05396-5] [PMID: 33550440]

[31]   Tindall LN, Xavier NA. Innovations in diabetes device training: A scoping review. Endocr Pract 2023; 29(10): 803-10. [http://dx.doi.org/10.1016/j.eprac.2023.05.012] [PMID: 37290557]

[32]   Zimbudzi E, Okada H, Funnell MM, Hamaguchi M. Editorial: Innovation in diabetes self–care management and interventions. Front Endocrinol (Lausanne) 2023; 14: 1269437. [http://dx.doi.org/10.3389/fendo.2023.1269437] [PMID: 37670874]

[33]   Majithia AR, Kusiak CM, Armento Lee A, *et al.* Glycemic outcomes in adults with Type 2 diabetes participating in a continuous glucose monitor-driven virtual diabetes clinic: Prospective trial. J Med Internet Res 2020; 22(8): e21778. [http://dx.doi.org/10.2196/21778] [PMID: 32856597]

[34]   Leksell J, Toft E, Rosman J, *et al.* Virtual clinic for young people with type 1 diabetes: a randomised wait-list controlled study. BMC Endocr Disord 2023; 23(1): 255. [http://dx.doi.org/10.1186/s12902-023-01516-x] [PMID: 37990315]

[35]   Prætorius T, Baymler Lundberg AS, Søndergaard E, Tang Knudsen S, Sandbæk A. The effect of virtual specialist conferences between endocrinologists and general practitioners about type 2 diabetes: study protocol for a pragmatic randomized superiority trial. Trials 2022; 23(1): 1059. [http://dx.doi.org/10.1186/s13063-022-06961-y] [PMID: 36578024]

[36]   Amdie FZ, Luctkar-Flude M, Snelgrove-Clarke E, Sawhney M, Balcha S, Woo K. Feasibility of virtual simulation-based diabetes foot care education in patients with diabetes in ethiopia: Protocol for a randomized controlled trial. Diabetes Metab Syndr Obes 2022; 15: 995-1009. [http://dx.doi.org/10.2147/DMSO.S345722] [PMID: 35386589]

[37]   Johnson CM, D'Eramo Melkus G, Reagan L, *et al.* Learning in a virtual environment to improve type 2 diabetes outcomes: Randomized controlled trial. JMIR Form Res 2023; 7: e40359. [http://dx.doi.org/10.2196/40359] [PMID: 36962700]

[38]   Vorderstrasse AA, Melkus GD, Pan W, Lewinski AA, Johnson CM. Diabetes learning in virtual environments: Testing the efficacy of self-management training and support in virtual environments (randomized controlled trial protocol). Nurs Res 2015; 64(6): 485-93.

[http://dx.doi.org/10.1097/NNR.0000000000000128] [PMID: 26505161]

[39]   Nerpin E, Toft E, Fischier J, Lindholm-Olinder A, Leksell J. A virtual clinic for the management of diabetes-type 1: study protocol for a randomised wait-list controlled clinical trial. BMC Endocr Disord 2020; 20(1): 137.
[http://dx.doi.org/10.1186/s12902-020-00615-3] [PMID: 32891126]

[40]   Seraj A, Mohammadi-Khanaposhtani M, Daneshfar R, *et al.* Cross-validation. handbook of hydroInformatics. Classic Soft-Computing Techniques 2022; Vol. I: pp. 89-105.

[41]   Xie J, Wang Q. A data-driven personalized model of glucose dynamics taking account of the effects of physical activity for type 1 diabetes: An *in silico* study. J Biomech Eng 2019; 141(1): 011006.
[http://dx.doi.org/10.1115/1.4041522] [PMID: 30458503]

[42]   Musuamba FT, Skottheim Rusten I, Lesage R, *et al.* Scientific and regulatory evaluation of mechanistic *in silico* drug and disease models in drug development: Building model credibility. CPT Pharmacometrics Syst Pharmacol 2021; 10(8): 804-25.
[http://dx.doi.org/10.1002/psp4.12669] [PMID: 34102034]

[43]   Kiani AK, Naureen Z, Pheby D, *et al.* Methodology for clinical research. Journal of preventive medicine and hygiene 632022;
[http://dx.doi.org/10.15167/2421-4248/jpmh2022.63.2S3.2769]

[44]   Ramspek CL, Jager KJ, Dekker FW, Zoccali C, van Diepen M. External validation of prognostic models: what, why, how, when and where? Clin Kidney J 2021; 14(1): 49-58.
[http://dx.doi.org/10.1093/ckj/sfaa188] [PMID: 33564405]

[45]   Patterson EA, Whelan MP. A framework to establish credibility of computational models in biology. Prog Biophys Mol Biol 2017; 129: 13-9.
[http://dx.doi.org/10.1016/j.pbiomolbio.2016.08.007] [PMID: 27702656]

[46]   Pollock RF, Norrbacka K, Boye KS, Osumili B, Valentine WJ. The PRIME Type 2 Diabetes Model: a novel, patient-level model for estimating long-term clinical and cost outcomes in patients with type 2 diabetes mellitus. J Med Econ 2022; 25(1): 393-402.
[http://dx.doi.org/10.1080/13696998.2022.2035132] [PMID: 35105267]

[47]   Duun-Henriksen AK, Schmidt S, Røge RM, *et al.* Model identification using stochastic differential equation grey-box models in diabetes. J Diabetes Sci Technol 2013; 7(2): 431-40.
[http://dx.doi.org/10.1177/193229681300700220] [PMID: 23567002]

[48]   Wilinska ME, Chassin LJ, Acerini CL, Allen JM, Dunger DB, Hovorka R. Simulation environment to evaluate closed-loop insulin delivery systems in type 1 diabetes. J Diabetes Sci Technol 2010; 4(1): 132-44.
[http://dx.doi.org/10.1177/193229681000400117] [PMID: 20167177]

[49]   Bellazzi R, Zupan B. Predictive data mining in clinical medicine: Current issues and guidelines. Int J Med Inform 2008; 77(2): 81-97.
[http://dx.doi.org/10.1016/j.ijmedinf.2006.11.006] [PMID: 17188928]

[50]   Mtshali S, Jacobs BA. On the validation of a fractional order model for pharmacokinetics using clinical data. Fractal and Fractional 2023; 7(1): 84.
[http://dx.doi.org/10.3390/fractalfract7010084]

[51]   Arlot S, Celisse A. A survey of cross-validation procedures for model selection. Stat Surv 2010; 4(none)
[http://dx.doi.org/10.1214/09-SS054]

[52]   McEwan P, Foos V, Palmer JL, Lamotte M, Lloyd A, Grant D. Validation of the IMS CORE diabetes model. Value Health 2014; 17(6): 714-24.
[http://dx.doi.org/10.1016/j.jval.2014.07.007] [PMID: 25236995]

[53]   Palmera AJ, Rozea S, Valentinea WJ, *et al.* Validation of the CORE Diabetes Model against epidemiological and clinical studies. Curr Med Res Opin 2004; 20(sup1) (Suppl. 1): S27-40.

[http://dx.doi.org/10.1185/030079904X2006] [PMID: 15324514]

[54]　Mackenzie SC, Sainsbury CAR, Wake DJ. Diabetes and artificial intelligence beyond the closed loop: a review of the landscape, promise and challenges. Diabetologia 2024; 67(2): 223-35.
[http://dx.doi.org/10.1007/s00125-023-06038-8] [PMID: 37979006]

[55]　Dankwa-Mullan I, Rivo M, Sepulveda M, Park Y, Snowdon J, Rhee K. Transforming diabetes care through artificial intelligence: The future is here. Popul Health Manag 2019; 22(3): 229-42.
[http://dx.doi.org/10.1089/pop.2018.0129] [PMID: 30256722]

[56]　Tasin I, Nabil TU, Islam S, Khan R. Diabetes prediction using machine learning and explainable AI techniques. Healthc Technol Lett 2023; 10(1-2): 1-10.
[http://dx.doi.org/10.1049/htl2.12039] [PMID: 37077883]

[57]　Roy M, Jamwal M, Vasudeva S, *et al.* Physicians behavioural intentions towards AI-based diabetes diagnostic interventions in India. Journal of Public Health
[http://dx.doi.org/10.1007/s10389-024-02235-w]

[58]　Phadke R, Prasad V, Nagaraj HC. Precise humane diabetes management: Synergy of physiological and psychological data in AI based diabetes. International Journal of Science and Technology Research 8

[59]　Walls M, Sittner K, Aronson B, Forsberg A, Whitbeck L, Al'Absi M. Stress exposure and physical, mental, and behavioral health among american Indian adults with type 2 diabetes. Int J Environ Res Public Health 2017; 14(9): 1074.
[http://dx.doi.org/10.3390/ijerph14091074] [PMID: 28926940]

[60]　Jia W, Fisher EB. Application and prospect of artificial intellingence in diabetes care. Medical Review 2023; 3(1): 102-4.
[http://dx.doi.org/10.1515/mr-2022-0039] [PMID: 37724106]

[61]　Wang SCY, Nickel G, Venkatesh KP, Raza MM, Kvedar JC. AI-based diabetes care: risk prediction models and implementation concerns. NPJ Digit Med 2024; 7(1): 36.
[http://dx.doi.org/10.1038/s41746-024-01034-7] [PMID: 38361152]

[62]　Borna S, Maniaci MJ, Haider CR, *et al.* Artificial intelligence models in health information exchange: A systematic review of clinical implications. Healthcare (Basel) 2023; 11(18): 2584.
[http://dx.doi.org/10.3390/healthcare11182584] [PMID: 37761781]

[63]　Aamer Mehmood M. Use of bioinformatics tools in different spheres of life sciences. J Data Mining Genomics Proteomics 2014; 5(2)
[http://dx.doi.org/10.4172/2153-0602.1000158]

[64]　Ponnarengan H, Rajendran S, Khalkar V, Devarajan G, Kamaraj L. Data-driven healthcare: The role of computational methods in medical innovation. Comput Model Eng Sci 2025; 142(1): 1-48.
[http://dx.doi.org/10.32604/cmes.2024.056605]

[65]　Grady C. Enduring and emerging challenges of informed consent. N Engl J Med 2015; 372(9): 855-62.
[http://dx.doi.org/10.1056/NEJMra1411250] [PMID: 25714163]

[66]　Qureshi R, Irfan M, Ali H, *et al.* Artificial intelligence and biosensors in healthcare and its clinical relevance: A review. IEEE Access 2023; 11: 61600-20.
[http://dx.doi.org/10.1109/ACCESS.2023.3285596]

[67]　Nie H, Zhang K, Xu J, Liao K, Zhou W, Fu Z. Combining bioinformatics techniques to study diabetes biomarkers and related molecular mechanisms. Front Genet 2020; 11: 367.
[http://dx.doi.org/10.3389/fgene.2020.00367] [PMID: 32425976]

[68]　Liu J, Zhang B, Zhu G, Liu C, Wang S, Zhao Z. Discovering genetic linkage between periodontitis and type 1 diabetes: A bioinformatics study. Front Genet 2023; 14: 1147819.
[http://dx.doi.org/10.3389/fgene.2023.1147819] [PMID: 37051594]

[69]　Dong Z, Lei X, Kujawa SA, Bolu N, Zhao H, Wang C. Identification of core gene in obese type 2 diabetes patients using bioinformatics analysis. Adipocyte 2021; 10(1): 310-21.

[http://dx.doi.org/10.1080/21623945.2021.1933297] [PMID: 34085602]

[70] Fernandez-Luque L, Al Herbish A, Al Shammari R, *et al.* Digital health for supporting precision medicine in pediatric endocrine disorders: Opportunities for improved patient care. Front Pediatr 2021; 9: 715705.
[http://dx.doi.org/10.3389/fped.2021.715705] [PMID: 34395347]

SUBJECT INDEX

A

Absorption variability 64, 70, 71
Accelerated recruitment 132
Accountability Act 106, 115
Accuracy 1, 2, 7, 48, 49, 56, 57, 83, 84, 92, 93, 111, 112, 113, 115
Adenosine monophosphate kinase (AMPK) 15, 16, 24
Adipose muscles 71
Advanced machine learning algorithms 133
Advancements in computational methods 3, 17
Agencies 103
Agonists 19, 20, 21, 22, 24, 25
AI-backed predictive analytics 125
AI-bioinformatics for improved prediction and personalization 125
AI-guided drug discovery 139
AI-powered clinical decision assistance 131
AI-powered models 137
Alogliptin 23
Alternative therapies 5, 64, 65, 68, 75, 77, 78, 112
Amino acid substitutions 25
Analysis of complex biological processes 4, 70
Application 1, 17, 65, 68, 72, 89, 127, 137, 138, 139, 140
Artificial Intelligence (AI) 1, 3, 7, 17, 55, 59, 125, 127, 131, 132, 136, 137, 140
Artificial pancreas 46, 47, 50, 51, 56, 65, 66, 67, 70, 71, 72, 78
Artificial pancreas systems 16, 46, 47, 59, 65, 85, 86, 88
Associated complications 11, 125
ATP channel 24
Audit Trails 105
Automated data analysis 132
Automatic therapy adjustments 129
Autonomy 99, 100, 101, 107, 108, 109, 118

B

Basal insulin rates 86
Beneficence 102
Benefits 21, 78, 84, 92, 100, 107, 108, 111, 114, 132, 136
Bias and Fairness in Models 111
Bifurcation Analysis Optimization Module 66
Biguanides 22, 23, 24
Binding Affinity Studies 21
Binding Site Identification 20
Binding Site Prediction 19
Bioengineering 125
Bioinformatics 66, 125, 126, 136, 138, 139, 140
Biological mechanisms 68
Biological systems 2, 5, 6, 17, 99, 102, 133, 136, 138
Biomarker Identification 138, 139
Biomedical health data analysis 68
Black-box models 111
Blood glucose levels 22, 24, 25, 49, 51, 53, 57, 72, 73, 77, 78, 89, 90, 91, 94
Blood Glucose Risk Index 94
Blood Pressure (BP) 14, 28, 52, 76, 77
Bolus doses 49, 84, 85, 87, 89, 90

C

Canagliflozin 23, 25
Candidate genes 23
Carbohydrate ratio (CR) 83, 85, 87, 90
Cardiovascular events 134
Chemical Reaction Engineering Module 66
Clinical data 71, 103, 104, 106, 112, 113, 114, 115, 130
Clinical Decision Support (CDS) 114, 115, 117, 129, 130, 137
Clinical Decision Support Systems (CDSS) 115, 130
Clinical endpoints 113
Clinical outcomes 110, 133, 134